I dedicate this book to everyone who has had to miss a workout session or stop exercising completely simply because of the inevitable time crunches that life brings.

Workout at Work™

Exercise Effectively Anywhere, Anytime Even at Work

Published by

MajorVision International

2017

Approved by The World Isometric Exercise Association

www.TWiEA.com

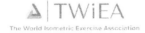

The World Isometric Exercise Association

www.MajorVision.com

Contents

Important General Safety and Health Guidelines

Important General Safety and Health Guidelines

This section entitled, Important General Safety and Health Guidelines, pertains to The ISOfitness™ Exercise System and team of people, the TWIEA (The World Isometric Exercise Association) and any association, collaboration, and partnership with TWiEA and any associated online resources, all print books and e-books, courses, publications, articles, videos, associated websites, recommendations, suggestions, coaching, advice either written, cyber, or verbal that is given, implied, or suggested, and all courses authored and/or delivered by Brian Sterling-Vete and Helen Renée Wuorio, the copyright holders, creators, writers, instructors, and the originators of the material including but not limited to The Bullworker 90™ Course, The Bullworker Bible™, The Bullworker Compendium™, The Doorway to Strength™, Feel Better in 70-Seconds™, Fitness on the Move™, Isometric Exercises for Nordic Walking and Trekking Pt 1 & 2, Improvised Isometric Exercise Devices (IIED) The Climber's Sling™, Improvised Isometric Exercise Devices (IIED) The Daisy Chain™, Isometric Power Exercises for Martial Artists™, The ISO90™ Course, Isometric Exercises for Golf Pt 1 & 2, The ISOmetric Bible™, Muscle Up for Menopause™, The Sixty Second Ass Workout™, The 70 Second Difference™, The TRISO90™ Course, TRISOmetrics™, The Zero Footprint Lockdown Workout™, and The Workout at Work™.

You should never begin any kind of sport, exercise system, workout plan, or diet modification, including everything contained in this book and any books mentioned in the beginning paragraph above unless you have consulted with and have the full approval of your medical doctor.

Your physician can accurately assess your current health status, and your ability to perform the exercises in the book and/or course. This is particularly important if you have any known or unknown pre-existing health issues, are pregnant, or believe that you may have other serious health conditions.

You must always have absolute approval from your physician before starting. Please show all the material in the above courses, books, video/audio, online material, and their content to your physician and get their approval before you start.

All exercises, suggestions, recommendations, instructions, exercise plans, dietary and eating recommendations, either given or implied or anything that falls under paragraph 1 is only intended as a reference source, and it is no substitute for a qualified professional personal coach to plan an exercise and diet program appropriate for your age and physical condition. Also, nothing mentioned in paragraph 1 is intended for use by children, and all exercise equipment must be kept out of their reach.

Never overexert yourself when performing any exercise. Stop exercising immediately and consult your doctor if you ever experience any pain, irregular heartbeat, shortness of breath, tightness in your chest/arms/fingers, faintness, nausea, or feelings of dizziness. Then consult your doctor and/or call the EMS immediately.

Always inspect any exercise equipment, and/or any/all other improvised or specifically made exercise equipment/materials, doors, door jambs, door frames, and anything else you use before each use to ensure its proper operation and to ensure that it is undamaged and safe. Do not use it unless all parts are free from wear, and it is functioning properly. Care should always be taken to avoid serious injury using any/all exercise equipment, and in all items, people, books, and courses mentioned in paragraph 1 of this section. Care should always be taken when getting into all exercise positions, on and off the floor, on and off chairs, on and off benches, on and off any other surface that might be used for exercise, including pieces of furniture, and in the use of all exercised equipment, either purpose-made or improvised.

No person, people, team, company, or organisation mentioned in paragraph 1 of this section can accept any responsibility whatsoever for any injury, harm, damage, illness, harm, damage to property, or any other negative health-related condition which may occur as a direct, or indirect result of following these courses, recommendations, suggestions, diagrams, pictures, videos, or while performing any exercises in these or any related other related material/publication/s.

For additional general information, we also recommend that you check reputable accredited medical advice sites such as The National Health Service in the United Kingdom, online at: https://www.nhs.uk/Livewell/fitness/pages/physical-activity-guidelines-for-adults.aspx

And: https://www.mayoclinic.org/healthy-lifestyle

Chapter 1: Time...

Time is a fascinating subject, and it has been debated, argued about, and studied since human beings first became conscious of the concept. It has been studied by scientists, religious leaders, and philosophers as they attempted to define exactly what it is and how it works. The greatest minds of the 20th and 21st centuries, including Professors Stephen Hawking and Albert Einstein, have pondered the infinite riddle that is time, with both making significant contributions to our understanding of time from a theoretical physics and cosmological perspective.

For most people, time is something much more basic. We are accustomed to thinking about time in terms of how linear time passes, and how that affects us. We also mark the passage of linear time with things like birthdays, taking holidays, and how long it will be before a special event such as a wedding happens, or perhaps a special anniversary. On a daily basis, most think about how many hours we must work each week to earn enough money to be able to pay our bills etc.

For people who exercise regularly, there are other aspects of time that have a great impact on daily life. These are things like calculating rest time between exercises, how long it takes to perform a specific exercise or workout session, and how a regular workout session can be made to fit into an already time-crunched schedule.

In this respect, the time factor can often be an annoyingly serious problem. This is because time, or rather the lack of time, is the number 1 reason why people either do not exercise or suddenly stop exercising regularly. Almost every survey about exercise and exercise habits reports the same results. This is that time is the most precious commodity we all possess, and it is the critical factor that determines success or failure when it comes to exercise, body shaping, and bodybuilding.

Time is a key advantage of performing advanced isometric exercises. This is because there is no faster way to exercise effectively to achieve the results you both want and need. Even if you are a professional-level athlete, the isometric system can still deliver the results you need, as fast, or even faster than via traditional methods.

Since spare time is often an extremely limited commodity for almost everyone today, it is not always going to be possible to maintain your regular gym visits when there are important time crunches in your life. If it is a virtual certainty that at some point you are going to be forced to miss your traditional regular gym session, then is it possible to improvise your workout in some way, so that it can still be done during your regular working hours? We believe that it is.

In this book, we are going to begin by examining exactly how much spare time you have, how much time is taken by exercising the traditional way in the gym, and how long it would take you to exercise effectively using the appliance of science with the isometric system to achieve the same results. Also, if it is possible and practical to exercise effectively at your place of work.

How Much Spare Time Do You Really Have?

To determine exactly how much spare time an average person really has available, as opposed to how much they think they have available, we will begin by looking at how much time we allot to various essential aspects of life in general on a daily, weekly, monthly, yearly, and even on a lifetime basis.

If we take the average life expectancy for someone in a modern Western country to be 80 years, then we can break everything down from there. Once the ineluctable time-consuming elements of life have been subtracted, we will see what is left at the end of it all.

Our starting point of 80 years breaks down into 960 months, or 29,200 days, or 4,171.42 weeks, or 700,800 hours. We all must sleep, and on average we spend $1/3^{rd}$ of our life asleep, which over a lifetime is 26.66 years, or 319.92 months, or 1,390.12 weeks, or 9,730.9 days, or 233,541.6

hours. This takes a huge segment removed from our lives, and when deducted it leaves just 53.34 years, or 640.08 months, or 2,781.3 weeks, or 19,469.1 days, or 467,258.4 hours left to live when we are awake.

If an average person spends just 3 hours a day watching TV, in a year that is 1095 hours, or 45.62 days. Whereas in a lifetime, it is 10 years, or 120 months, or 521.42, weeks, or 3,650 days, or 87,600 hours. After deducting the amount of time that the average person spends watching TV during their lifetime from their overall life expectancy, it leaves just 43.34 years, or 520.08 months, or 2,259.87 weeks, or 15,819.1 days, or 379,658.4 hours left to live. Thinking about this in perspective, it certainly makes one think twice about habitually spending hours each day watching junk TV, mostly filled with brainwashing advertisements. With a little effort and imagination, it is always going to be possible to find something better to do with your increasingly scarce commodity, time.

Almost everyone must work, and if our working life is between 20 and 65 years of age, this is a 45-year/540-month period. During that period, if the working week is an average of just 40 hours, and it is often much more, then this is 2,080 hours or 86.66 days of non-stop work in a year. This is 10.68 years, or 128.2 months, or 556.88 weeks, or 3,898.2 days, or 93,556.8 hours in a 45-year working lifetime. This then leaves only 32.66 years, or 391.92 months, or 1,702.99 weeks, or 11,920.9 days, or 286,101.6 hours left to live.

Commuting to work takes a significant amount of time each day, and most people have an average of 7 years, or 84 months, or 365 weeks, or 2,555 days, or 61,320 hours over a working lifetime. This then leaves only 25.66 years, or 307.92 months, or 1,337.99 weeks, or 9,365.9 days, or 224,781.6 hours left to live.

Spending quality time with your family and loved ones is critical, and central to who we all are as people. However, mostly due to work-life restrictions, the average time spent with family and loved ones is only an average of about 8 hours per week. This is 416 hours a year, or 33,280 hours, or 3.79 years, or 45.58 months, or 198.09 weeks, or 1,386.66 days in a lifetime. This then leaves only 21.87 years, or 262.34 months, or 1,139.9 weeks, or 7,979.24 days, or 191,501.6 hours left to live.

If you now factor in regular exercise via traditional methods for only 3 days each week, involving an average 1-hour gym session, then this adds up to a total of 3 hours a week, or 12 hours a month, or 156 hours a year. Or 12,480 hours, or 520 days, or 74.28 weeks, or 17.09 months, or 1.42 years in a lifetime. This now leaves just 20.45 years, or 245.25 months, or 1,065.62 weeks, or 7,459.24 days, or 179,021.6 hours left to live.

However, the 1-hour gym portion of a regular workout is not all that is involved for most people. The problem is that you currently cannot "beam" instantly into the gym to begin your workout session, therefore, you must factor in several other integral components. These are the elements of travel time to and from the gym, time spent finding a parking space once you are there (often during peak periods) and changing room/shower time both before and after your gym session. If you now add the time taken for these unavoidable elements, then it can easily add an extra 2 hours to your 1-hour gym session, making it a total of 3-hours for your overall exercise-devoted time.

Therefore, 3 hours a day should be factored in as the time that is devoted to exercise and exercise-related matters.   3 hours a day, 3 times each week makes a total of 9 hours. 9 hours a week is 468 hours a year, or 19.5 days a year, or 34,440 hours, or 1,560 days, or 222.85 weeks, or 51.28 months, or 4.27 years in a lifetime. This then leaves only 17.6 years, or 211.06 months, or 917.05 weeks, or 6,419.24 days, or 157,061.6 hours left to live.

Even at a basic exercise level, this is not an insignificant part of your overall life that you are devoting to exercising, and exercise-related matters, especially when it is becoming increasingly clear to see just how scarce and valuable your time is.

However, if you are serious about exercising to improve your sports performance, or if you just love to exercise, then this whole equation must be dramatically re-calculated.

Instead of settling for an exercise session on 3 days each week, you will probably increase this to 5 days a week, Monday to Friday, and typically after work as you travel home. Since we have already established that you cannot instantaneously "beam" yourself into the gym, all the other unavoidable elements of travel time, traffic problems, searching for parking, changing time, and showering must still be added. 5 hour-long sessions of exercise in a gym each week must be tripled to become an average of 15 hours that is being devoted exclusively to exercise, and exercise-related matters weekly. 15 hours a week, is 780 hours, or 32.5 days each year, which is 62,400 hours, or 2,600 days, or 371.42 weeks, 85.47 months, or 7.12 years in a lifetime.

Therefore, if you exercise the traditional way in a gym for 5 days each week, when you have added in all the inescapable elements that come with it, this leaves you just 14.75 years, or 176.87 months, or 767.58 weeks, or 5,379.24 days, or 129,101.6 hours left to live.

Whichever way you look at it, devoting that much time to exercise is extremely significant. It is a massive chunk out of any daily, weekly, monthly, and yearly schedule. More importantly, it is a life-changing amount of time taken out of your life that can never be recovered. Obviously, you cannot exercise continuously for 7.12 years, so, if we take an average 9-hour working day as the entire time spent exercising each day over that same period, then this becomes much more.

Inconvenient Truths About Gyms, Gym Memberships, Exercise Classes and Personal Coaches

It is just an indisputable fact that most people do not want to exercise, and therefore, never do any. If they did, then not only would there be many more gyms, fitness classes, and personal coaches everywhere, but the general population of Western countries would be much healthier and in better physical shape. The statistics about gyms and the fitness industry, in general, speak for themselves. Research stated by Noobgains.com indicated that in the United Kingdom, around 4.5 million adults are gym members, which is only about 7% of the population, and in the United States 14% of the population are gym members, which is around 45 million people. In both countries, those who enjoy exercise enough to be gym members represent a mere fraction of the overall population, with the remaining people mostly doing little or nothing. A survey by Hustle in 2019 found that 63% of gym memberships go completely unused, and 82% of gym members go to the gym less than once per week. The Global Health and Fitness Association, IHRSA, reported that the annual attrition rate for gyms and fitness clubs is 28.6%. More importantly, 22% of people completely stop going within six months of starting their membership, and a little over 31% of people admit that they would have never spent the money in the first place had they been able to predict how little they would use the facility.

Even the best intentions fall short every year with 4% of all New Year's resolutions being broken by the end of January and 14% by the end of February. This is a problem for the gym industry because about 12% of all new gym memberships are bought in January and 80% of those who join at that time have quit within 5 months (source: 2012 Coupon Cabin). In general, and not simply because of a New Year's resolution, according to IHRSA, 50% of all new gym members quit within 6 months, and 46% of the former gym members reported that they quit because of gym membership costs.

Of those people who do exercise, the majority report that they do not particularly enjoy doing it and given a choice they would prefer not to. However, most people know that they must do some exercise for their health, so it is a real dilemma. Taking an overview of the situation combined with spare time being such a precious commodity, one can begin to understand why virtually all fitness campaigns have failed over the years. The problem is further compounded because most coaches and gyms recommend exercise sessions and methods that are time-consuming and require certain specialist equipment. When it comes to people who do not particularly enjoy regular exercise or those who are only doing it because they know they should, then they are typically being recommended to perform the type of exercise that they will almost always give up on.

This is ironic and counterproductive, and it continues to compound the health and fitness problems for the majority of the population. It makes no sense whatsoever, except for commercial reasons because gyms and personal coaches want to tie their clients into continually needing their services rather than provide a practical long-term solution. Why gyms and personal coaches do this always baffles us because in many ways they are selling their new customers a product and service that the end-user does not want and it is not even practical for most in the long term Since gyms and personal coaches are highly unlikely to retain these people as customers, then it would be refreshing for them to recommend something practical such as isometrics and focus their efforts on the people who enjoy exercise. This means that gyms, health/fitness centres, and personal coaches who take this approach are actually part of the greater overall problem of why most people do not exercise regularly.

Since we know what most people want from an exercise system, which is maximum output for the bare minimum input, then why not give it to them instead of selling them something they do not want and will either rarely or never use? This is why the isometric exercise system and the Workout at Work™ concept provide the ideal solution. In many ways, it could be described as being a scientifically proven exercise system for people who do not like exercise. However, for those who do enjoy exercise and do it to a high level, isometric exercise is a way to develop great strength and muscle size.

Moreover, since time is so precious for most people, and those who do not like exercise and yet still do want to spend the minimum time and effort doing it, the isometric exercise system is the perfect solution. Is the isometric exercise system the perfect system for everyone? No, it is not. However, no other single exercise system is perfect either. Does the isometric exercise system deliver excellent results in a short space of time, and is it scientifically proven? Yes, it certainly does and is.

More importantly, a properly performed isometric exercise takes so little time to do, and in its most basic form requires no equipment whatsoever, the system can easily be incorporated into an average working day. Also, those who are exercising this way are typically completely unnoticeable because the system is so subtle and discrete.

For those who enjoy exercising and love their gym memberships, I am not for one moment suggesting that the exercises they do are not worthwhile, because they are excellent. However, the isometric system is time-efficient and a great tool to use on busy days. This is not an either-or dilemma, it is about keeping an open mind when it comes to embracing new, equally effective methods. Besides, I do not think that anyone on their deathbed will reminisce and think, "I wish I'd spent more time in the gym instead of with my family/wife/loved ones." If someone does, then they are probably delirious.

For some, exercise in a gym can become a total obsession. When this point has been reached, exercise die-hard types will completely structure their entire life around having access to a suitable gym at least once a day. This obsession can become so severe that the repercussions can affect every aspect of their family life, usually for the worse.

For example, it can make family holidays and special events far less enjoyable and memorable, and it can make travel away from home, and from the local gym that they love so much almost impossible. I have even seen some exercise die-hard types become extremely stressed during a simple discussion about having to travel away from home, and the gym, for business or family matters.

Thankfully, most people who exercise regularly, are not obsessed with it to this extent. However, many people can still become frustrated and irritated if they cannot build in enough time each day to complete a regular workout routine. Even without the die-hard obsession factor regarding exercise, the time constraints of modern life still typically cause problems, irritations, and stress for exercise enthusiasts. The point I am making is that people can very easily develop tunnel vision in their preferred type of exercise.

Once they start on a journey down this tunnel, then these people quickly become convinced that the only effective form of exercise that exists and works, is the exercise routine that they follow with the equipment they use in the local gym. Once this point has been reached, then for them, nothing else exists. At that point, it is almost heresy to suggest that there may be other forms of exercise that work equally well, and perhaps better than their beloved system. Some people can even become extremely defensive if alternative suggestions are made.

If you have found a system of exercise that works well for you, then that is great. We suggest that you stick with it, and enjoy the results you get from it, and the experience you have while exercising. However, you should also remember that a change is as good as a rest, especially when it comes to exercise. Even if you have what you believe to be the perfect system of exercise, one that surpasses all else, then it still does not mean that you will not eventually find something else that can work equally well.

More importantly, if you keep an open mind, then you may find something that will work so well that you can effectively substitute it, to replace your much-loved gym-based exercise routine. This new alternative system could be a highly effective complement to your weekly routine/system, especially if you can use it effectively while you travel away from home for either business or pleasure.

Chapter 2: Workout at Work

New research has revealed beyond doubt, that your office job is damaging your health, especially if you sit at a desk for more than 6 hours a day. Dr Allan Stewart, MD, Director of Aortic Surgery, Icahn School of Medicine at Mount Sinai, stated in a recently published article that sitting for long periods caused a lowered heart rate, and that caused other serious problems.

People who work for long periods at a desk tend to eat snacks, and fast food, which is less nutritious than whole foods. Your muscles burn less fat simply because you are not active, this lack of activity encourages an increase in the circulation of fatty acids and cholesterol to the heart. The result is an increased risk of a heart attack.

Research has shown that even if you exercise 3 or 4 days each week after work, it is not enough, and it will not fully offset the damage caused by sitting at a desk for 6 hours a day or more.

Sitting at a desk for more than 6 hours a day increases your insulin resistance. Being less resistant to insulin is linked to type 2 diabetes. Unless you are physically active for even just a short time during every 30 to 60-minute period, then you will gain excess fat around your waist. This is because you are not processing glucose enough, and therefore, you will gain fat.

The latest research has also shown that even if you are highly active over the weekend, serious damage will already have been done during the week through comparative inactivity while working at your desk. Regular breaks to do something physical every hour, or half-hour, during the working day are essential to good health, and weight control.

Long periods working at a desk each day will also increase your risk of injury. This is because inactivity will cause strength loss in key muscles and muscle groups. Poor posture is a side effect of weakened musculature due to long periods of seated deskbound work each day. A major side-effect of poor posture is the restricted oxygen intake due to forward bending shoulders.

The simple fact is that a compromise must be found. One that enables people who must sit for long periods each day at a desk to work, and one that keeps employers happy because there is no productivity loss associated with even a short period of physical activity.

Therefore, the isometric exercise system is the perfect solution. In our assessment of how much time we either must or voluntarily devote to the basic elements of life, we have established that our daily work takes up a huge amount of the time we have available to us.

We have already covered the basics of time, and exercise. We know that time is the number 1 reason why people either do not exercise or suddenly stop exercising. We know that time is one of the most critical and scarce resources each of us has. We also know that advanced isometric exercises are either as effective or often more effective than a traditional gym-based resistance workout session.

Integrating exercise sessions into your working day should be essential, and actively encouraged by business leadership. This is because there are a great many more benefits to productivity, alertness, creativity, illness prevention, and overall efficiency than there are downsides to the slight loss of time taken out of the working day.

In relation to your work, regular exercise has an enormously positive effect. Exercise improves the way you generally feel because you release endorphins, and because exercise causes your brain to release serotonin, it helps to beat anxiety and depression. This combination makes you feel happier and makes work and life-related stresses easier to handle. The result of this improved state of mind has a positive effect on your work and your work relationships with colleagues.

Improved wellness is another huge benefit of regular exercise. It reduces the risk/probability of developing certain cancers, increases your ability to fight illness, improves your heart and cardiovascular efficiency, and reduces the risk of developing type 2 diabetes.

Some research has even indicated that if you are doing a sedentary job, then doing something physical regularly every 30 minutes can make you up to 30% more efficient at your work. What employer would not want their employees to be working at maximum efficiency? If you are self-employed, then surely you need to always be at the top of your game and work at maximum efficiency.

If the "something physical every 30 minutes," were exercises that lasted for several minutes or more, and disrupted people working around you, then it would be entirely understandable if employers refused to let it happen. However, what if there was no disruption to others whatsoever? What if each exercise lasted for just 7 seconds? Surely that would make it a complete "no-brainer" to incorporate 1 exercise every 30 minutes as a part of a standard working day for all employees.

The isometric exercise system allows you to do exactly that, and to exercise quickly and effectively while you are at work. You do not have to try and create time during your lunch break to slot in a traditional gym-based workout if you have the luxury of a long enough lunch break. With the isometric system of advanced isometric exercises and a pair of Iso-Bows®, you can even perform a high-intensity pro-level total-body workout session without even leaving your desk. This is because the system of exercises requires what we call a Zero Footprint Workout™ environment. If you can stand up, and/or sit down, then this is enough space to perform a total-body workout. More importantly, you do not even need to use up any of your precious lunchtime breaks, which is especially important if you are not allowed much time.

If you work an average 9-hour day, and if you perform one 7-second exercise while you are at your desk every 30 minutes, then at the end of your working day you have completed an 18-exercise total-body workout routine. The 18 exercises have only taken 126 seconds to perform, or 2 minutes and 6 seconds out of your working day. This is much less time than an average person will take out of their working day for basic bathroom breaks.

Just 126 seconds of exercise time, spread out in 7-second bursts every 30 minutes, will have a hugely positive impact on the quality of your life, and your work. imagine that at the end of each workday, you have not only enjoyed a more productive day whatever business you are in; you have also completed a high-quality total-body workout. This then means that you can go straight home, out socially, or do whatever you want. The important thing is that you do not have to spend almost all evening at the gym (or performing matters related to that,) or just get home late and probably miss saying goodnight to your kids (if you have any,) before going straight to bed.

Interestingly, since the isometric requires no movement, it is very discrete. Most people who were observing you perform a 7-second exercise, would not even realise that you were exercising. Instead, the most common thought people have about isometric exercises is that from an observer's perspective, they could easily appear to be nothing more than stretching exercises. This suggestion is reinforced by the exercise time of 7 seconds. Even if a 10-second isometric exercise were performed, then to an observer it would still appear that you were doing nothing more than stretching.

Stretching is something that everyone does several times throughout each day, especially when sitting at a desk for long periods. The only thing that would be slightly out of the ordinary would be that from an observer's perspective, some sort of stretching strap was being used, AKA the Iso-Bow™. This makes the isometric exercise system, and the Iso-Bow™ perhaps the ultimate form of stealth exercise technology. They enable you to exercise virtually anywhere, at any time, and without overtly appearing to be exercising or to be performing a full workout routine. Zero Footprint Workout™ workouts and stealth exercise technology that even have the capability of delivering a pro-level high-intensity workout is quite an advance from noisy, time-consuming, equipment-reliant, and expensive traditional exercise systems.

The isometric exercise system gives you back your life, and it gives you total exercise freedom in a way that no other exercise system can.

Chapter 3: Alternative Exercise Methods

There are several methods of exercise that are viable and satisfactory alternatives to a traditional gym-based exercise routine. The first that comes to mind is a basic freehand callisthenic routine. A callisthenic routine simply means bodyweight-only exercises of various kinds, such as push-ups, pull-ups, squats, lunges, trunk curls, and dips etc. The word "callisthenics" is derived from a combination of the ancient Greek words "kalos," which means "perfect," and "sthenos," meaning "strength."

These exercises are excellent at building and maintaining levels of high levels of fitness, balance, endurance, and a considerable degree of strength. Certain callisthenic exercises can develop great strength, such as the ones used by gymnasts. These are primarily pull-ups, dips, and handstand dips. During the gymnastic-style exercises, the gymnast performing them would adjust the speed, velocity, and angles that the exercise is typically performed, which usually significantly increases their difficulty. These exercises almost always include a portion of isometric, or static, exercise hold as well.

There is a serious drawback to advanced callisthenics being a complete substitute for a gym-based strength workout. This is because for most people without gymnastic skills, once you have become accustomed to handling your body weight when performing the various exercises, then you need to use techniques to place you at a biomechanical disadvantage to gain increased resistance.

In addition, you need a certain degree of equipment available, and/or similarly improvised facilities to allow a gymnastic-style workout routine to be performed. At the very least, you will need equipment or facilities to perform pull-ups and dips. If you do not have these, then unless you find another way of applying more resistance through biomechanical disadvantage during each exercise, you are primarily only performing a basic fitness/resilience/endurance routine. You are almost certainly not performing a resistance routine that is focused on growing strength and muscle.

The other major drawback is that you need a certain degree of space to perform an effective gymnastic-style callisthenics workout routine. Therefore, you cannot perform any exercise easily, and relatively unobtrusively in a public or semi-public place. Instead of callisthenics, is there another alternative and effective way to exercise? An exercise method that delivers similar, or often even greater benefits than traditional weight training as a gym does. An exercise system that takes much less time to perform and that can be performed almost anywhere. An exercise method that only requires the bare minimum of equipment and that uses quite possibly the world's most compact total-body gym that can easily fit into your pocket.

Yes, there is a practical and effective solution. The isometric system is a method of advanced exercise that does exactly that. Each exercise takes between just 7 and 10 seconds to perform, and it only requires two small pieces of equipment.

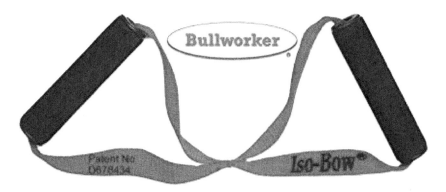

The exercise equipment we recommend is an Iso-Bow®. Even a pair of them are so compact that they can easily fit into the average jacket pocket or jeans pocket, they can easily fit into a handbag, an average purse, or a briefcase.

More importantly, with a pair of Iso-Bows®, you can effectively exercise every major muscle group of the body. The level of workout you can get from using a pair of Iso-Bows® can range from an easy, low-level beginner's workout, right up to a very high-intensity professional athlete level of workout.

Amazingly, you can do all of this without any adjustment being needed to the Iso-Bows®. Each user will benefit proportionately, according to the amount of effort and force that is applied during each exercise.

A simple 7-exercise workout routine, such as one from "The 70 Second Difference" book, will exercise every major muscle of the body in a single session. More importantly, it will only take between 49 and 70 seconds of consecutive exercise time to perform if you take no break whatsoever between exercises. This is not typically possible for most people, however, even factoring in a full 1-minute break-time between each exercise, adding a total of 7 minutes of rest time to the overall workout still means that your total-body exercise session will be completed in between only 7 minutes and 49 seconds/469 seconds, or 8 minutes and 10 seconds/490 seconds if you are taking your time.

As you get fitter, or if you are already fit when you start the exercise routine, then the amount of rest time taken between exercises can be dramatically reduced. It can easily be reduced by 50% or more. In fact, there is no reason why someone who performs this workout regularly, should not be able to reduce the amount of rest time between each exercise to between only 10 and 20 seconds. This makes it easily possible to perform the complete total-body exercise routine in as little as only 110 seconds, or 1 minute and 50 seconds.

Even with long rest periods factored in, there is still a considerable amount of time that is saved by using the isometric exercise system, especially when compared to traditional methods of gym-based exercise. The realistic projections for how much time already physically fit people would save by comparison are astonishing.

For example, let us take an advanced athlete, or a sports professional, who suddenly faces an unavoidable time-crunch situation. They can still benefit from a professional gym-level workout routine with the isometric exercise system. Even when exercising at the very highest levels of intensity, it still will not take long to complete a total-body workout. Furthermore, the isometric workout can be performed almost anywhere relatively unobtrusively. So, even professional athletes can still get a high-level total-body workout no matter where they are, even while travelling as a passenger in a car, on a train, or a plane. The result? The workout is not missed, and the time crunch is resolved.

How Much Time Can an Isometric Exercise Workout Save?

The isometric exercise system can save an enormous amount of time. It can reduce your daily total-body workout routine to somewhere between 5 and 10 minutes in length. Many people who do not know about, or do not fully understand exercise science are naturally sceptical and find this hard to believe.

However, when people learn about the masses of hard science that support these claims, and about the effectiveness of brief, focused, and highly intense exercise sessions, then they soon become converts. The isometric exercise system is all about following the science because following the science gets results faster than most people believe possible. The isometric exercise is about not confusing activity with accomplishment in relation to exercise, as most traditional exercise systems do.

For example, let us examine how a high-level exercise enthusiast, a semi-professional, or even a professional athlete would use an isometric exercise workout routine, and how long it would take them to perform it.

Taking a comprehensive 20-exercise workout, with each exercise being performed at more than one position along the Range of Motion (ROM) of each joint/limb produces a total of 40 exercises to be performed during the routine. If each exercise is performed with the highest level of force possible for the recommended 7 seconds per exercise, this gives a total of 280 seconds, or 3 minutes and 40 seconds, of consecutive exercise time.

Since this example is about someone who is already fit, they would not require a long rest period between exercises. We know that muscle has a recovery half-life of about 3 seconds after stopping an exercise, so, after just 9 seconds the muscles will be ready for the next exercise. Therefore, to be generous we will add 10 seconds of rest time between each of the 40 exercises. This now gives a total of 680 seconds, or 11 minutes and 20 seconds needed to complete the entire workout routine.

Performing an effective high-intensity professional-level isometric workout in only 11 minutes and 20 seconds a day is nothing short of amazing. More importantly, it is a real option for you right now. Unlike most other systems, you do not need a gym to perform isometric exercises, or any expensive exercise equipment because your Iso-Bow® total-body gym can easily fit into your pocket. You also do not need to waste money on gym memberships, and you will save hours of valuable time in your first month alone.

Let us see how much time you can save using the isometric exercise system, and how this can impact your life. If you exercise 3 times each week using the isometric system, it will take a very generous absolute maximum of 680 seconds, or 11 minutes and 20 seconds a day, for 3 days each week. This is 2,040 seconds, or just 34 minutes of exercise a week.

The traditional method of visiting a gym each evening to exercise on your way home from work would take an average of 9 hours each week. This means there is already a massive time saving of 8 hours 26 minutes in your first week of performing the isometric exercise system. Exercising the traditional way over a year would take 468 hours/19.5 days. Exercising using the isometric exercise system over a year would take just 1,768 minutes, or 29.46 hours, or 1.22 days.

This is a massive time saving of 438.54 hours or 18.27 days in a year. You have a choice of either exercising using the isometric exercise system for just over 29 hours spread out over an entire year, at virtually no cost, and with no restrictions in respect of where you can exercise, or you must devote a massive 468 hours/19.5 days a year, you will need a fully equipped gym, plus a lot of money in gym membership fees, transport, and parking charges etc., to achieve similar results.

Next, we will take someone who loves to exercise and might be committed to building serious strength and muscle. This type of person would probably perform 5 workout sessions each week at a gym. Therefore, we will examine how much time would be saved by using the isometric exercise system to achieve similar results.

Using traditional gym-based methods, exercising 5 sessions each week will consume a considerable 15 hours a week, or 780 hours a year. This is a massive 62,400 hours, or 2,600 days, 85.47 months, or 371.42 weeks, or 7.12 years of your life that you will spend in a gym.

Using the isometric exercise system would take only 56 minutes a week. This is a mere 2,912 minutes, or 48.53 hours, or 2.02 days each year. This is just 3,878.4 hours, or 161.6 days, or 5.31 months of exercise over an entire lifetime.

The isometric exercise system will save you an incredible 58,521.6 hours, or 2,438.4 days, or 80.16 months, or 6.68 years of your life. Just imagine what you could do with an additional 6.68 years of life. Imagine for one moment that you were terminally ill, and near death. Suddenly, a miracle happens, and you could get an additional 6.68 years immediately added to your life expectancy. How would you choose to spend that additional time? Would you choose to spend the entire 6.68 years of your extended lifespan in a gym? Instead, perhaps you would prefer to spend that time travelling to see more of the world, having fun, and/or spending that precious time with your loved ones. In short, generally do things that are more enriching for your soul. I wonder what your honest answer to that question is...

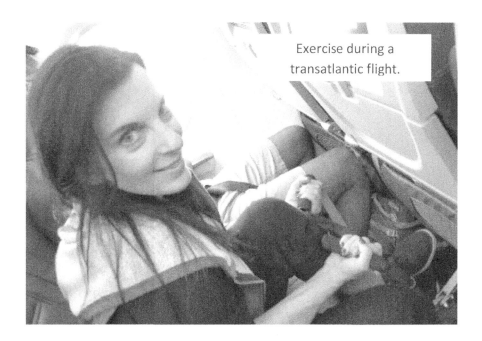

Exercise during a transatlantic flight.

The Zero Footprint Workout

Isometric exercises, even when performed at a high level of intensity, which a professional-level athlete would perform would require little space. An isometric exercise workout can be performed in what we call a zero-footprint exercise environment. This means that if you can stand up, or sit down on a chair or bench, then you can perform a total body workout without needing any additional room.

With the isometric system, you can exercise effectively at work in the office, at home, while travelling as a passenger in a car/train/plane, or on the beach during your summer holidays, the choice is yours. You are never going to be restricted by needing to have a gym nearby, and you do not need to waste a fortune on gym membership fees either. You are set free to build and shape the body you want, in almost no time, and for almost no cost.

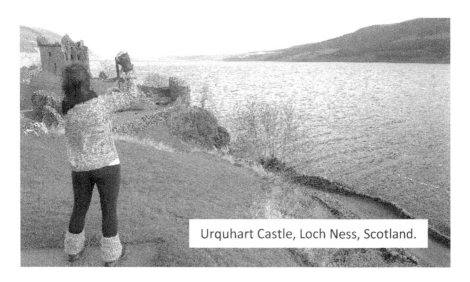

Urquhart Castle, Loch Ness, Scotland.

Using the isometric exercise system we have benefitted from gym-standard, high-intensity exercise sessions while on transatlantic flights, on high-speed rail trips, as car passengers on road trips, on board a ship crossing the Mediterranean, on the ramparts of the famous Urquhart Castle on the banks of Loch Ness in Scotland, during a break from fell

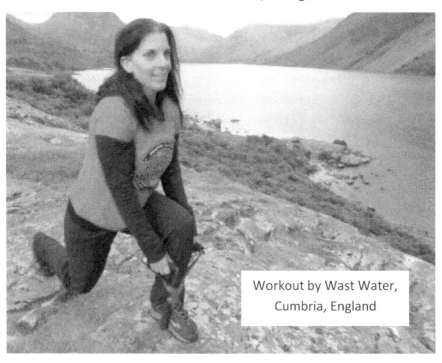

Workout by Wast Water, Cumbria, England

walking around Eskdale and Wast Water in the English Lake District, during several TV outside broadcasts while working with a famous US TV network, and on the remote beaches and rocky coves in Cornwall, England.

We may have occasionally turned a few heads and attracted the attention of people who were nearby while we were exercising. However, almost all the attention was focused on how simple and effective isometric exercises were.

For those who want to become fit, very strong, and grow serious muscle, while at the same time leading a very busy lifestyle, working long hours each day/week, travelling away from home a lot for business or pleasure, or for people who simply have better things to do than spend most of their life in a gym, then the preferred method of exercise is obvious.

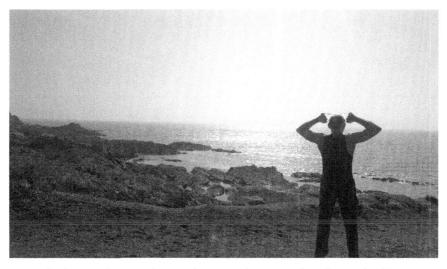

An isometric exercise workout on the coastal path overlooking Holywell Bay Beach, Cornwall, England, while the TV show Poldark is being filmed.

Chapter 4: Exercise Science Overview

In this section, we will give a user-friendly overview of exercise science together with the features and benefits of various exercise techniques and concepts. For those who want more in-depth information about the science of isometric exercise and health and fitness in general, then we suggest that you also read our books The ISOmetric Bible™ and The 70 Second Difference™ books. Both are available on Amazon.

The Basic Types of Resistance Exercise

All muscle training falls into between two or three specific categories, depending upon how you break them down. In the most basic form, there are two types, either contraction with movement, or contraction without movement. Breaking them down a step further there become three categories, with one being isotonic, another isokinetic. Last but certainly not least, is isometric.

Isotonic training is all about movement with muscle shortening and lengthening during the lifting and lowering phases of the exercise. We know that the isotonic category can be broken down further into three parts. One part is the concentric contraction, which is the lifting phase of an exercise when the muscles shorten. Another is the eccentric phase which is the lowering part of an exercise when the muscles lengthen.

Lastly in this isotonic category is the isokinetic contraction. This is where the muscle changes in length during both the concentric and eccentric phases of the contraction, however, the velocity remains constant no matter how much force is applied during the exercises.

Then comes the isometric category. With an isometric exercise, there is no movement whatsoever. To help you envision this, I will take a random weight training or freehand callisthenic exercise such as a chest press because it can be performed either with movement OR without movement, as an isometric exercise.

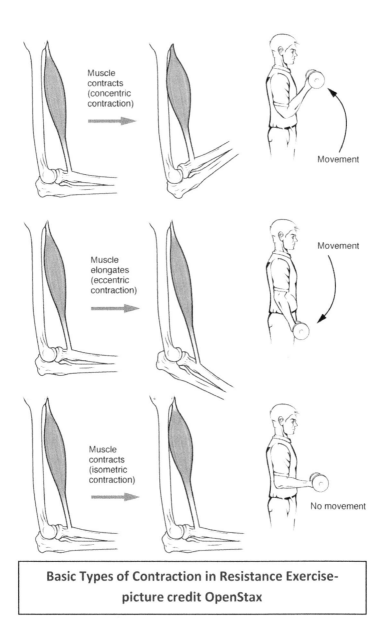

Muscle contracts (concentric contraction)

Movement

Muscle elongates (eccentric contraction)

Movement

Muscle contracts (isometric contraction)

No movement

Basic Types of Contraction in Resistance Exercise-picture credit OpenStax

For example, a barbell, a machine, or your bodyweight can be lifted and lowered to perform an exercise such as a barbell curl, this is called, isotonic exercise, callisthenics or simply exercise with movement.

To perform the same or similar exercise isometrically you would attempt to perform the same or similar biomechanically correct actions of a barbell curl, however, at a certain point, or points if multiple exercise points were being used, the curling movement would stop because an immovable object point had been reached.

At that point or points, you would apply an increasing level of force until you reach the desired target level as you attempt to perform the curling exercise against the immovable object.

At the desired isometric exercise point, a constant force is applied against the immovable object for 7 seconds which is the optimum isometric exercise time. The ideal basic isometric exercise point for general exercise is roughly at the mid-point when your muscles reach a stalemate working against each other or an immovable object. This is called a Standard isometric Contraction.

The harder you engage your muscles as you try to break the stalemate by lifting, pushing, or pulling, the stronger your muscles become. In doing so, you engage many more muscle fibres than normal as you attempt to move the immovable object and perform the curling exercise action.

Doors, desks, chairs, walls, and many other everyday items work well as immovable objects BUT the easiest and most used immovable object is typically yourself.

Isometric Overview

As you now know, isometric exercise does not involve any movement. Instead, the joint angle and the muscle length do not change during contraction. You also now know that 7 seconds is regarded as the optimum time to perform an isometric exercise.

However, almost everyone when exercising tends to count the exercise elapsed time much faster than real elapsed time. This means that it is easy not to reach the magic 7 seconds of the optimum isometric exercise time. Therefore, we always suggest aiming to perform the exercise for 10 seconds to ensure that the 7-second target is always reached even when under the stress of performing intense exercise.

Isometric exercise has been extensively scientifically researched and has been proven time and again to be a highly efficient way to build great strength and grow muscle. In fact, isometric exercise is probably one of the most thoroughly researched of all exercise systems. However, it also remains one of the most misunderstood systems of exercise. This is almost certainly through fear, professional ignorance and purely financial reasons.

Several different techniques can be used in the isometric exercise system. Most of these techniques are highly advanced for use by competitive athletes, competitive martial arts practitioners, strength athletes and bodybuilders. Therefore, they have no application as part of a general isometric exercise session for the average person who simply wants to get generally stronger and fitter.

However, purely out of interest I will list them here, and in case any fitness enthusiasts, athletes or bodybuilders read this book and wish to try them. They are described in greater detail in our book called The Isometric Bible which is available on Amazon and in good bookstores. The most common and advanced isometric exercise techniques include the following:

- △ Standard Isometric Contraction
- △ Yielding Isometric Contraction
- △ Maximum Duration Isometrics
- △ Oscillatory Isometrics
- △ Impact Absorption Isometrics
- △ Explosive Isometrics, AKA: Ballistic Isometrics
- △ Static-Dynamic Isometric
- △ Isometric Contrast
- △ Functional Isometrics
- △ TRISOmetrics™

There are more than enough isometric exercises that can be performed without any equipment whatsoever to allow a total body workout routine to be completed relatively easily. These will typically be self-resisted isometric exercises, which are excellent. However, by using only minimal readily available equipment such as walking poles, golf clubs, martial arts belts, climbing ropes, scuba diving webbing weight belts, and broom handles etc. it is possible to greatly expand the number of exercises that can be performed.

It is also perfectly possible to adapt and use other readily available items such as tow ropes, steel chains, towels, and commonly found immobile objects such as sturdy fixed barrier railings, solid walls, solid doors, door frames, or parked vehicles to perform a complete isometric exercise routine. Again, these are all excellent improvised exercise tools that allow an expanded range of highly effective isometric exercises to be performed.

Using improvised exercise tools can yield an unexpected additional benefit. This is because it allows one to focus more and apply greater concentration to each exercise. This is particularly useful for those who are either completely new to, or who are relatively new to the isometric exercise system. We will explain more about what these can be later in the book.

One of the things we love about both the isometric and self-resisted systems of exercise is that as you get stronger through exercise, you can apply more force and overall intensity to your isometric or self-resisted exercises.

This, in turn, means that you can gradually increase the level of force you can safely apply to each exercise which will mean that the results and benefits you receive will grow in a compound way through regular daily use. This is what we call a natural Adaptive Response™ mechanism which is a useful aspect of our biology.

Isometric Exercise Science

Even until the mid-20th century, there was almost no scientific research that had been performed into the benefits of isometric exercise. We also know that before the first serious scientific research study, how people trained isometrically was typically by performing what we now call endurance isometrics.

Thankfully, isometric exercise has now been thoroughly scientifically researched and proven for several decades. I would estimate that there has probably been at least as much scientific research performed into isometric exercise as there has been into traditional resistance training.

The first major in-depth study into isometric exercise was performed at the world-famous Max Plank Institute in Dortmund, Germany. If you already have a reasonable knowledge of science, you will also know that the Max Plank Institute is a world-renowned centre of scientific excellence in many disciplines.

Between 1953 and 1958, one of the most extensive research studies was commissioned into isometric exercise science. These experiments are now considered by many to be the original gold standard of isometric exercise studies. The results were made widespread public knowledge in the resultant ground-breaking book, The Physiology of Strength, by Dr Theodor Hettinger - Research Fellow at the Max Plank Institute. During that 5-year research period, Dr Hettinger and Dr Muller performed a widely reported, reputed 5,500 experiments, although this figure is almost certainly apocryphal because they would have had to perform a minimum of three experiments a day, every day for five years. Research suggests that the actual number of experiments performed by Hettinger and Muller was probably closer to 200, however, in wider studies at other institutions since that time, over 5,500 studies have almost certainly been completed. These were conducted on male and female volunteers from all walks of life, and at every level of strength, fitness, and athletic ability. Perhaps what surprised people the most was how dramatic and impressive the results were gained from performing isometric exercises. Also, because the same or similar results were easily repeatable it made the data gained from the experiments exceptionally reliable.

The conclusion of the extensive studies proved beyond doubt the overall superiority of isometric exercise when it comes to building both strength and muscle, compared to traditional isotonic exercise methods. It also proved that the isometric system delivered these results much faster and with far less exercise than traditional resistance training. Another extremely interesting result emerged from the experiments. This was because it was not the length of time that an isometric exercise was held that produced the optimum results. Instead, it was the correct level of force applied for a very specific optimum time. They found that performing only one daily isometric exercise for between just 6 and 7 seconds, and at only two-thirds of an individual's maximum effort, could increase strength by an average of up to 5% per week. By any standards, strength gains of 5% in exchange for the expenditure of only 66%, or around two-thirds of an individual's maximum capacity, is an excellent result.

Perhaps even more amazingly, they discovered that after someone has performed a single 7-second training stimulus (exercise) per day, the muscle being exercised in that same position was no longer responsive to further gains. In other words, it did not matter how many more times you exercised the same muscle in the same position, there would be no further increase in muscle growth or strength. The only way to do this was to perform another isometric exercise at a different position only the ROM (Range Of Motion) of the limb being exercised. The scientific data about this can be referenced on pages 28 to 31 of Dr Theodor Hettinger's book, "The Physiology of Strength."

In 2001, Nicolas Babault PhD of the University of Burgundy, Dijon, France, led a team of scientists to research and examine how many muscle fibres were activated, and how long they remained active during both traditional weight training and isometric training.

45

(The scientific research paper is published: Nicolas Babault, Michel Pousson, Yves Ballay, and Jacques Van Hoecke - Groupe Analyse du Mouvement, Unite´ de Formation et de Recherche Sciences et Techniques des Activite´s Physiques et Sportives, Universite´ de Bourgogne, BP 27877, 21078 Dijon Cedex, France.)

They discovered that when training intensely, and in near-perfect style, the levels of muscle activation during repetitions of optimum maximal weight training were between 89.7% during the concentric contraction, or when lifting a weight, and 88.3% during the eccentric contraction, or when lowering a weight. For practical purposes, an average of about 89% overall.

The study also revealed that during the lifting, or concentric part of the exercise, the maximum intramuscular tension only lasted for between 0.25 and 0.5 seconds. Which, for practical purposes is an average of about 1/3rd of a second during each isotonic repetition.

This is because traditional isotonic resistance exercises naturally involve movement. They also have aspects of velocity and acceleration to consider in the overall equation. "Force" is only produced for a split second, to produce a maximal contraction of the muscle fibres.

The same research also showed that the level of muscle activation during isometric exercise was as high as 95.2% and that it lasted for the entire 7 to 10 seconds of each exercise. This is a huge increase over the 1/3rd of a second muscular activation achieved during a single repetition of weight training.

Therefore, based on these discoveries, technically a single isometric exercise performed at only two-thirds of an individual's overall maximum can deliver either similar or often even better results, than the equivalent of up to 3 sets of 10 weight training repetitions in the lifting phase of the exercise.

To explain this further I will use a typical barbell curl exercise in the lifting phase as my example, where the object of the exercise is to engage as many muscle fibres as possible in a maximum muscular contraction. Naturally, 3 sets of 10 repetitions give us an overall total of 30 repetitions. One set of 10 repetitions of the barbell curl in perfect high-intensity style produces a total maximum muscular engagement for a total of approximately 3.3 seconds. Three sets of 10 repetitions of the same exercise, a total of 30 repetitions will result in a total of approximately 9.9 seconds of maximum muscular engagement, and an average of 89% muscle activation overall.

In comparison, one high-intensity isometric contraction exercise produces a maximum muscular engagement that lasts for the entire duration of the exercise. Even though the optimum time over which an isometric exercise is performed was found to be 7 seconds, this is almost always rounded up to the 10-second target number. The maximum muscular engagement will last for the entire 10 seconds of a high-intensity isometric exercise and with 95.2% muscle activation overall.

This is proof that is based entirely on scientific research that 3 sets of 10 near-perfect high-intensity curls when weight training, which takes several minutes to perform, were still not equal to the results achieved by a single 10-second high-intensity isometric curl exercise.

The Standard Isometric Contraction

The standard isometric contraction is a simple and highly effective technique. Therefore, this is the technique we will focus on for practical isometric training.

The standard isometric contraction, AKA: overcoming isometric contraction, AKA: maximum-effort isometrics, or whatever else you wish to call it, is when a muscle is applying force to push or pull against an immovable resistance. This is the most basic of all kinds of isometric exercise, and it is highly effective.

This type of isometric contraction exercise was performed during the experiments by Dr T. Hettinger and Dr E. Muller at the Max Plank

Institute. It is also the technique referred to in their book "The Physiology of Strength".

In a standard isometric contraction, it is theoretically possible to exert up to 100% of one's maximum capacity effort against an immovable object and then continue to hold that level of force throughout the exercise.   This means that standard isometric contraction can be a very high-intensity exercise system.

Performing an isometric exercise against an immovable object at a certain level of force for a given duration of time will teach your body to recruit more muscle fibres to try to move the object. As you perform the exercise and generate as much force as possible, your CNS, or Central Nervous System, learns that it needs to activate and recruit more muscle fibres to reach the goal of moving the object.

Since this will naturally be impossible to move, the process will continue each time you exercise to make you stronger and grow more muscle. Your body mechanisms become trained to readily activate and recruit additional muscle fibres as needed when facing repeated similar challenges, which in turn, repeats the cycle more readily every time.

As we mentioned earlier, the immovable/solid object that is used can be anything that is completely solid and completely safe to use. This can be a wall, a door, a door jamb, a parked motor vehicle or anything similar. Perhaps the most common objects used to enhance everyday isometric exercise training are sturdy towels, climbing ropes, martial arts belts, scuba diving weight belts, webbing straps, golf clubs, and broom handles etc. All the aforementioned items are excellent when used properly, and all will deliver some excellent results. More importantly, they are typically readily available for most people which makes exercising with them so much easier.

Another common way to perform isometric exercise is to do it in a self-resisted way. Self-resisted means that you push or pull against your limbs, hands, and feet etc. For example, you might place the palms of your hands together at chest level with your hands roughly at the midpoint of your body. In that position, you would then press your hands together using your chest muscles to provide the primary driving force. Suddenly, you are performing a highly effective self-resisted isometric chest exercise!

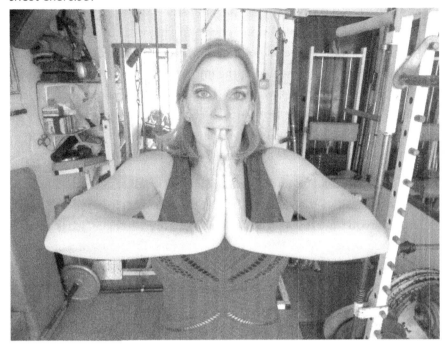

It is possible to perform a well-balanced and highly effective self-resisted isometric workout to exercise virtually every section of the body. So, never underestimate self-resisted exercise because it can be immensely powerful indeed. Also, self-resistance exercises are an excellent way to ensure that a personal maximum resistance is used safely, and with minimum risk of injury caused by applying too much force. The fact is that it does not matter which method is chosen. It can be isometrics performed against an immovable object, self-resisted isometrics, or a combination of the two. The most important thing is that either the object must be completely immovable through human muscle power alone, or the force of one body part must be able to completely counterbalance the force of another body part to produce a muscular stalemate.

Intensity, Force, Strength, and Power

Intensity is always going to be a relative term, and it is often completely misunderstood when it is used concerning exercise. When it comes to exercising your muscles, the intensity is the % of your ability to move a resistance. Technically, an individual's highest possible level of intensity is when they reach a point of momentary failure after exerting themselves completely. However, the important questions we need to try and find answers to are: "How hard is hard?" and "How intense is intense?" To some degree, both are very subjective things. Taking two people of roughly equal fitness, something that is intense to one person might be considered comparatively easy to the other.

Hard is a relative term, and handling 50 lbs of resistance is impossibly hard if your strength is only at the level required to lift 49 lbs. However, if you can lift 100 lbs as a maximum, then lifting 50 lbs is going to be comparatively easy. Often, the only factors differentiating between people and the intensity level exerted, are going to be mental toughness, determination, and perception. Therefore, to gain the greatest benefits from isometric exercise the first thing that must be learned is how to determine, with a reasonable degree of accuracy, what level of intensity is being applied to an exercise. It is just a fact that what one person deems to be 100% of their capacity will always be quite different from another person's estimate. The accurate estimation of what one person deems to be 2/3rds of their overall maximum force will also vary from person to person. The accuracy of estimation will also vary greatly between an experienced professional athlete and an absolute beginner to exercise.

Experience has taught us that most people who are new to exercise will always fall well short of accurate estimation of any given percentage. A beginner will find it more challenging to accurately estimate what 2/3rds of their 100% maximum is when compared to a more experienced athlete. Many people might believe that they are performing at 100% capacity when they are only performing at around 2/3rds, or even perhaps at just 50% or less of their 100% maximum. This is because exercise is new to them, therefore, the experiences and feelings in their body which are associated with it are also new. They simply have no common frame of reference when it comes to calculating/estimating their level of physical exertion.

The human brain has a built-in mechanism that helps to protect the body and prevent it from performing a physical activity to such a level that could cause serious damage or even death. This is the mechanism that makes your brain tell you to stop exercising when it begins to get tough, and the feeling of wanting to stop exercising only increases as you continue to push yourself harder to do more. This is all despite the biological fact that you are physically capable of doing much more than is being suggested by the messages you are receiving from yourself.

Over time, the brain of people who exercise regularly, and especially to a high level of intensity, will naturally adjust, and reposition this built-in safety margin. This means that the brain of an experienced high-level athlete does not "tell" them to stop an exercise until the level of intensity is much higher than it would be for a beginner. Therefore, when it comes to exercise, how is it possible to subjectively quantify, and then impart appropriate levels of recommended intensity? This problem is made even more challenging when one considers the fact that accurately translating and subjectively assessing various levels of intensity will, to some degree, always be subjective to every individual.

If you were to train as hard as humanly possible, with near 100% maximum intensity which involves super-strict form, and training to complete failure and beyond, then you simply cannot train for a long time. It is just physiologically impossible. Physics and biology are quite simple in this respect. The intensity of your workout is directly proportional to the length of time that you are physically able to perform your workout. The harder and more intensely you exercise, the shorter time that you will be physically able to perform the exercise. Make no mistake, performing a 7-second isometric exercise while exerting close to your personal 100% maximum physical capacity is completely and utterly exhausting, even for a professional athlete.

What does all this mean when it comes to accurately communicating to another person various levels of exercise intensity, especially when there is no professional coach or elaborate and expensive measuring equipment at hand? Research clearly shows that almost everyone will stop exercising long before they are in any danger of becoming seriously fatigued. Most people will *think* they are achieving a much higher level of intensity than they would if they were only a little more mentally resilient.

This does not mean that people should suddenly begin pushing themselves beyond their physical limits, which would be a stupid thing to do. However, it does mean that most people who enjoy a higher-than-average level of mental resilience and determination, as well as being in physically good condition, can push themselves much harder than they might think. If anyone ever feels "genuine" strain or fatigue to the point of becoming injured, then they should stop exercising immediately. Even without the aid of a professional coach to monitor, encourage you and measure your progress with specialist equipment, the tips we have outlined in this section will help you to get the most out of every workout. It is also worth remembering that if you cheat, then the only person who loses is "you."

As a footnote, for the sake of clarification. Exercise intensity refers to how much energy is expended when exercising which includes the amount of weight used per repetition, and Perceived intensity varies with each person. Intensity and force are technically different but are frequently accepted as interchangeable terms in the common vernacular. Muscular strength is different from muscular endurance, which is the ability to produce and sustain muscle force over a certain period of time. While strength is the maximum force you can apply against a load, power is proportional to the speed at which you can explosively apply it. In other words, it is the ability to produce a given amount of force quickly. Muscular force, often referred to as muscular strength, is the physical power exerted by muscles to perform various actions, such as lifting, pushing, or pulling objects. It results from the contraction of muscles and is vital for human mobility and functionality.

Technically, How Does a Muscle Grow?

How does a muscle grow? This is one of the most common questions asked concerning fitness and exercise in general. However, it is also one of the most misunderstood concepts, even amongst fitness professionals and personal trainers. To see for yourself just how uninformed or badly informed some people are, simply join one or two of the social media groups online so you can read some of the absolute drivel posted by 'keyboard warriors' who purport to be 'experts' on the subject. Alarmingly, many of these people seem to have developed a hardcore following, which to the science-based professional is like watching 'fools leading other fools' on a wild goose chase.

So, back to the key question which is, how does a muscle grow? To explain this, we must examine three concepts, which are: 1) muscle growth through increases in the volume/size of myofibrils inside the muscles, which is commonly called myofibrillar hypertrophy. 2) hyperplasia, which is when there is an increase in the number of muscle cells/fibres. 3) sarcoplasmic growth which is all about increasing the fluid content.

When it comes to the subject of exercise, the muscles you wish to grow must be challenged with a workload that is greater than they can currently accommodate. In other words, an exercise that is intense enough to stimulate growth. This stimulus can come from any source such as lifting a heavy object, weight training, isometrics, compressing a spring in a device such as a Bullworker™, or through self-resistance either hand to hand or limb to limb or using an Iso-Bow™ etc.

This process creates trauma to the muscle fibres which disrupts the muscle cell organelles. This then triggers other cells outside the muscle fibres to greatly increase in numbers at and around the point of the trauma to repair the damage. The process of repair involves a fusion of cells. This, in turn, causes the cross-sectional area of the muscle fibre to increase because the muscle cell myofibrils increase in both size and quantity. This process is more commonly known as hypertrophy. Since this process increases the number of cellular nuclei the muscle fibres generate more myosin and actin. These are contractile protein myofilaments which in turn help to make the muscle stronger.

This is the basis of what is more commonly known as myofibril muscle growth. In addition to this, there is also probably a process called hyperplasia which takes place. I use the term, 'probably' because this concept is extremely controversial for many reasons. One of the key problems is that evidence of this in human beings is lacking, whereas there is a mass of evidence supporting hyperplasia in mice and other animals.

Hypertrophy is the increase in the size of the existing muscle fibres to accommodate the increased demands placed upon them through intense exercise. Hyperplasia, concerning skeletal muscle growth, is the increase in the number of muscle fibres which in turn will also increase the cross-sectional area of a muscle.

Despite there being a lack of evidence supporting hyperplasia in human beings, logic supports the process taking place. This is because of a theory known as Nuclear Domain Theory. This states that the nucleus of a cell (a muscle cell in this instance) is only able to control a finite area of cellular space. It is thought that satellite cells donate their nuclei to the muscle cell until a certain point is reached whereby this can no longer take place.

Beyond a certain limit, and through continued intense training, the cell must eventually divide to create two cells instead of the former single cell. When this happens, the entire hypertrophy process starts over once again. This probably means that most of the muscle growth is almost certainly caused by hypertrophy, and a much smaller percentage can be attributed to hyperplasia at any given point in the muscle stimulus/growth process.

Finally, there is a subject of sarcoplasmic muscle growth to address. Sarcoplasmic muscle growth is the increase in the volume of sarcoplasmic fluid in the muscle cell. These are the fluid and energy resources surrounding the myofibrils in your muscles containing mostly glycogen together with other elements including creatine, ATP, and water etc.

To clarify, glycogen is simply a type of sugar that serves as a form of energy. It is deposited in bodily tissues as a store of carbohydrates, and it is the body's main form of storage for the sugar, glucose. Glycogen is stored in two main places in the body, one being the liver, and the other being the muscles.

More importantly, glycogen is the body's secondary source of long-term energy storage, with the primary energy storage source being fat. When glycogen is in the muscles, it is converted into glucose for use as energy when performing sports etc., and glycogen stored in the liver is converted into glucose for use as energy throughout the body, and in the central nervous system.

Therefore, sarcoplasmic growth increases muscle volume, but this increase is not in functional strength mass since it does not increase the number of muscle fibres. It is like 'the pump', in that it is an increase in the size and shape of the muscle through the muscle holding an increased amount of fluid.

Rest Time Between Exercises

Naturally, the rest time taken between exercises during a workout is quite different from the rest and recovery needed to recover and allow your body to positively respond to the stimulus generated by exercise.

If you keep the rest time between exercises brief enough, then the workout routine itself will give you an excellent cardiovascular workout, and this is what we recommend that you ultimately aim for. If you are already very fit, then we would recommend that instead of performing the optional cardio routine you simply put more effort, force, and overall intensity into each isometric exercise. At the same time, aim to keep the rest time between those exercises as brief as possible. This approach will help you work towards being able to perform each exercise so that it has an Ultra-High Intensity Ultra-Short Burst™ effect, which will greatly improve your overall fitness level, and boost your Base Metabolic Rate or BMR.

However, if you are not already fit, then to begin with you may wish to simply allow each isometric exercise to deliver all the cardio you need as you gradually build up your levels of fitness and endurance. Eventually, you will increase your level of fitness to a point where you can begin to gradually reduce the rest time between each exercise to a minimum point that works best for you.

Once you have learned how to fully engage the muscles during each exercise with sufficient force, and at the same time, you have learned how to breathe fully, deeply, and naturally throughout each exercise. At the same time, you should be keeping the rest time between exercises to a minimum because this combination will have an excellent and beneficial cardiovascular effect.

Dynamic Flexation™

Dynamic Flexation™ is a technique we devised to help ensure that we gained maximum benefit from the isometric portion of our exercise regimens. I will recap and briefly summarise the Dynamic Flexation™ technique as originally laid out in "The 70 Second Difference™" book.

We always recommend that everyone who performs any kind of resistance exercise practices some form of Dynamic Flexation™ before performing any exercise. This will help to ensure that all muscles, tendons, ligaments, joints, and your spine have become naturally and properly engaged in the correct biomechanical exercise position.

We would never recommend that as soon as you assume an exercise position you should suddenly apply maximum power and force right away. This is unless you are a very experienced athlete, or unless you are training with a qualified coach to perform a certain type of isometric exercise to develop extra power such as a static-dynamic or explosive/ballistic isometric technique. Instead, we recommend that you always breathe naturally as you gradually flex and engage your muscles and joints into performing the exercise.

To perform Dynamic Flexation™ you gradually flex your grip and the muscles you are about to exercise while applying an increasing level of force immediately before performing the exercise. The exercise is then performed, and to disengage from the exercise we recommend reversing the Dynamic Flexation™ engagement process.

Our preference is to apply tension and force to the exercise gradually through Dynamic Flexation™ typically for between 2 and 3 seconds, or even for as long as 4 seconds if needed. This all takes place before beginning to count the required 7-second exercise time of the isometric contraction.

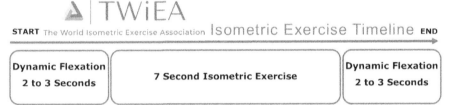

We prefer using one deep full breath in and out as a method of more accurately counting each second that has elapsed. This way, you will time each exercise more accurately, and you will not be tempted to hold your breath at any point which is a mistake that beginners often make.

Similarly, at the end of an exercise, we do not recommend that it be ended abruptly. Instead, we recommend reversing the Dynamic Flexation™ technique so that you gradually relax as you slightly move each muscle and joint out of the exercise position.

This process helps enormously because when you are in a good position it will help you to gain the maximum benefit from each exercise you perform. Dynamic Flexation™ is when you move and adjust your feet, legs, hips and especially your hands as you gradually assume a solid

57

position and handgrip. As you flex and move, you will be making micro-adjustments.

All exercises will be performed best if you assume a correct and solid handgrip, fist clench, or foot position etc. One of the most important aspects of assuming the correct exercise position begins with your grip. Without a solid grip on a bar, handle, or anything else you need to hold while exercising, you will naturally be setting yourself up to perform sub-maximally. You can also be helping to develop injuries which can include sore elbows, joints, ligaments, and tendons.

Dynamic Flexation™ is a concept that embraces the broader principles of motor unit recruitment, and "Henneman's Size Principle" to increase the contractile strength of a muscle. Elwood Henneman's principle stated that under load, the motor units in a muscle are engaged according to their magnitude of force output, from the smallest to the largest, and in task-appropriate order.

This means that the slow-twitch, low-force, fatigue-resistant muscle fibres are activated before any fast-twitch, high-force muscle fibres are engaged which are less fatigue-resistant. Since the body naturally works in this way, it enables precise and finely controlled force to be delivered at all levels of output.

This also means that when exercising, or when performing tasks in daily life, the fatigue which is experienced as a result will always be minimised. It will also be proportional to the sequential engagement of the most appropriate muscle fibres being engaged.

Isometric Exercises and Blood Pressure

Some exercise critics point out the fact that when someone performs an isometric exercise it will raise their blood pressure. However, the same people also very conveniently forget that the same is also true of all other forms of exercise including freehand callisthenics and traditional isotonic resistance training with weights.

All physical activity, and especially exercise will cause your blood pressure to rise for a short time. Providing that you are in good health, it is important to always breathe deeply, naturally, and normally when performing any exercise, then any rise in blood pressure will soon return to a normal level when the exercise is stopped. The faster this happens, the fitter you are.

For those who are advanced athletes and/or are used to hard and intense isometric training for a long time, you will already have made significant progress in strengthening your heart and circulatory system.

For those who are new to isometric training, just like with any form of exercise, the best way into it is by taking it slowly and less intensely at first.

Newcomers to exercise, and especially isometrics, should always focus on applying less force, to begin with, and on always breathing fully and deeply throughout all exercises. NEVER HOLD YOUR BREATH!

Under strict medical supervision, even those with Coronary Artery Disease and high blood pressure should be able to increase their physical activity levels with a reasonable degree of safety. However, if you are a person who already suffers from high blood pressure, then you should always exercise at a much lower level of intensity than someone who has no physical issues.

Furthermore, **EVERYONE, ESPECIALLY PEOPLE WITH HYPERTENSION, OR ANY FORM OF CARDIOVASCULAR DISEASE, SHOULD ALWAYS CHECK WITH THEIR DOCTOR BEFORE BEGINNING ANY KIND OF EXERCISE ROUTINE**.

Rest and Recovery

When calculating your ideal recovery period, many things must be taken into consideration. These include your age, your current health and fitness level, the quantity of exercise taken, and most importantly the intensity of the exercise which has been performed.

Some people will need a recovery period of between 24 and 48 hours, and for others, the recovery period may be as brief as between 12 and 24 hours.

As a rule, the recovery period will always incrementally increase as the intensity of the exercises increases towards an individual's 100% potential maximum capacity. Always be aware of this and make sure that you factor this into your rest and recovery time calculations. The diagram will help to outline this.

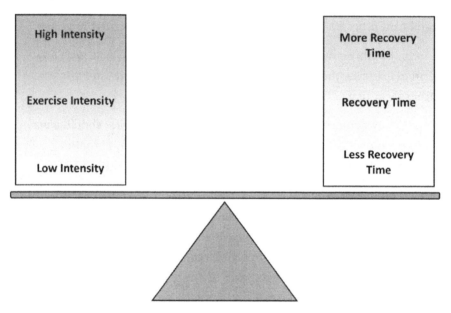

Sports scientist J. Atha's research revealed something remarkable. This was that when performing isometric contraction exercises at two-thirds of an individual's maximum capacity, the average person could safely perform an exercise like this daily, without overtraining.

Standard isometric contraction exercises can be safely performed daily, by almost anyone, of almost any age, and in almost any physical condition as a means of strength development, body shaping, and even bodybuilding.

However, for more intense workouts, we recommend a full rest day between workouts due to the higher demands being placed upon the

Central Nervous System (CNS) and the time needed to fully recover and benefit from the exercise. Several other factors affect post-exercise recovery. These include a balanced and properly executed stretching routine and getting enough quality sleep. While you sleep, your body releases certain hormones which help you to repair and rebuild damaged tissue, and which will directly help your muscles to grow.

Adequate Nutrition is Vital

Quality post-exercise nutrition will help your body repair itself faster, decrease your recovery time, and help to maximise the benefits gained from the exercise. Research shows that post-exercise immunodepression peaks if you exercise for longer than you are currently capable, and problems are enhanced due to reduced or inadequate nutrition. Hydration is also one of the most important factors in your recovery, as well as for your overall health, especially since your muscles are mostly composed of water. Early studies suggested a 30 to 60-minute window after exercise when you need to eat, after which, your body begins to draw upon itself to repair and recover from your workout. Later studies found that this window can be anything from 1 to 3 hours depending on the workout type, overall intensity, and goals. On average, since most leave 60 minutes after food before hard exercise, and if a workout lasts an average of 45 minutes, then a 30 to 45-minute window to eat after exercise will mean it has been up to 150 minutes (2.5 hours) since your last food, therefore, the earlier suggested 30–45-minute window still makes sense for most people especially if they want to build more muscle and strength.

Most people mistakenly consume excessive amounts of protein at the expense of other key nutrients such as carbohydrates. Therefore, in doing this they are working against their best interests and overall optimum health. One of the key nutrients that have been found to help enormously when in recovery from prolonged periods of heavy exercise is carbohydrates. A lot of research supports the hypothesis that carbohydrate is the most important nutritional factor in preventing post-exercise immunodepression. Most do not realise that the protein composition of human muscle is typically only somewhere in the region of between 18/9% and 21% protein (average 20%) and the rest is made up of water, glucose, lipids, and carbohydrates etc. We will not go into more detail here, however, if you want to learn more about this and many other surprising nuggets of useful information about sensible nutrition and exercise then they can be found in 'The 70 Second Difference' book.

Strength, Stamina, Endurance, and Resilience

It is important to understand the difference between strength, stamina and endurance because once understood, you will then be able to devise the most suitable workout routines according to your body type.

Muscular strength is possibly best understood as being a muscle's capacity to exert force against resistance, or weight. This is comparatively easy to measure because your ability to lift a given amount of weight for a single repetition is a good measure of your strength.

Stamina is the length of time at which a muscle, or group of muscles, can perform at or near its maximum capacity. For example, the number of squats you can perform with a given weight which is 90% of your maximum would be a measure of your stamina or the overall distance that you can carry a similarly heavy object such as an anvil.

Endurance is all about time, and your ability to perform a certain muscular action for a prolonged period regardless of the capacity at which you are working.

Resilience is all about your ability to recover from whatever stresses and demands are placed on your muscles. However, resilience is mostly all about your state of mind, your mental toughness and ability to endure, perform and deliver under pressure, and how you recover quickly emotionally.

The muscular composition of your body will always determine how well you will perform in certain sports. The amount of slow twitch muscle fibres you possess will determine how well you perform at endurance-related events, and both type A and type B fast twitch muscle fibres are all about explosive power and your ability to maintain it.

In simple terms, if you possess mostly slow twitch fibres, then you are naturally going to be better suited to endurance sports. Alternatively, if you possess mostly fast twitch muscle fibres, then you are a natural weightlifter. It is important to note, that no matter what your natural predisposition might be in this respect, with the correct training regimen, it is still possible to significantly increase your abilities in your naturally weaker opposing areas of speciality.

The TRISOmetric™ Exercise Concept

The TRISOmetric™ exercise concept was first developed in the mid-1980s by Brian Sterling-Vete as a high-intensity method when he was training with 4-times World's Strongest Man Jon Pall Sigmarsson in Iceland. He wanted to dramatically increase the training intensity without simply increasing the weight we were lifting and reducing the rest time between. Then weight increases would follow at the newly elevated level of base intensity.

The TRISOmetric™ exercise can be performed with any type of resistance equipment, however, it does not necessarily need a gym or gym equipment in order to get a good workout session. It is perfectly possible, and to many people preferable, to perform a TRISOmetric™ exercise workout using self-resisted isometric exercises or a range of simple IIEDs or Improvised Isometric Exercise Devices.

These can comprise readily available items such as a climbing rope, a doorway pull-up bar, or a towel. The TRISOmetric™ exercise technique can also be performed very easily with a Bullworker®, Steel Bow®, Iso-Bow®, and/or Iso-Gym®, or a combination of all the above. The Iso-Bow® is our preferred exercise device of choice, preferably a pair of them.

The TRISOmetric™ exercise system is a combination of three scientifically proven techniques into a single unified approach. These are as follows.

- ▲ Level 1 – Single Position Isometric Exercise.
    - ○ Isometric exercise is proven to be more efficient at building strength and muscle than traditional isotonic exercise.
- ▲ Level 2 – Triple Position Isometric Exercises.
    - ○ Dividing the ROM (Range Of Motion) into three segment points of roughly equal distance, and then performing an isometric exercise at each point, will deliver even muscle-building and strength gains across the entire ROM of the limb being exercised.
- ▲ Level 3 – Combine Super-Slow Isotonic Exercise with level 2.
    - ○ Super-slow isotonic exercise delivers better gains in muscle size and strength than performing the same exercise faster. Super-slow exercises engage more muscle fibres for longer.

The system also incorporates other scientifically proven aspects including a specific length of time taken between each exercise, and Ultra Short Ultra High-intensity bursts of exercise etc. Since isometric exercise is one of the most efficient and result-producing in terms of the ratio of the effort expended and results gained.

In practice, to perform one complete set of a TRISOmetric™ exercise, firstly, a single isometric exercise is performed in each of three positions along the ROM (Range Of Motion) of the body part being exercised. Each of the isometric positions chosen will divide the range of motion of the limb roughly into three equal parts. This way a more even strength curve is developed for the muscle being exercised. This takes advantage of the strength gain overlap area of + and – 20% around the point of the isometric exercise chosen. However, more equally divided isometric exercise positions can be employed by more advanced practitioners.

Next, the focus is on rest time. There must be no longer than 10 seconds of rest time between each isometric exercise. Once all three (or more) isometric exercises have been completed, then once again with a maximum rest time of just 10 seconds, an appropriate isotonic exercise is performed to exercise the same muscles or muscle group. The isotonic exercise can be performed with either a Bullworker®, a Steel Bow®, an Iso-Bow®, and Iso-gym®, as freehand callisthenics or with weights/resistance machines.

It does not matter what equipment you use, or if you use any equipment, or not. The correct execution of the corresponding exercise is what is most important. The isotonic portion should be performed in a super-slow style. This means that each repetition should take 10 to 12 seconds to perform in the concentric or lifting phase where the muscles shorten, and another 10 to 12 seconds to perform in the eccentric or lowering phase where the muscles lengthen.

If you perform each portion of the TRISOmetric™ exercise correctly, then you will find it extremely intense. We recommend that you do not attempt to repeat the exercise again and that you do not perform any other exercise for the same muscle/muscle group. The fact is that if you perform the TRISOmetric™ exercise correctly you will probably NOT be able to or indeed have any desire to perform more. it is all about focus, force, overall intensity, and the quality of what you do, and not about the quantity.

During the experimental phase as I developed the TRISOmetric™ exercise concept, I concluded that it was better for the CNS, or Central Nervous System, to perform the isometric phases first. The data I gathered from several research papers clearly indicated that this made each isometric exercise more effective while at the same time minimising overall negative stress.

The maximum 10-second rest period is just enough to allow the muscle being exercised to almost recover before the next exercise is applied. Naturally, this will place a high demand on the cardiovascular system of anyone performing this system. Therefore, if this is an issue, either increase the rest time and/or reduce the level of applied force and overall intensity during each isometric exercise accordingly. The objective would then be to gradually improve by decreasing the rest time between exercises while increasing the level of force that is applied. Eventually, your overall fitness level will increase to allow you to perform higher-intensity exercises during each phase of the TRISOmetric™ exercise set you are performing.

Never be tempted to perform more sets because this can be counterproductive. If you feel the need to do more, then it is always better to apply even greater force to each isometric exercise while decreasing the speed of the already super-slow portion even more.

As a general guide, if you feel that you can perform another set of the TRISOmetric™ exercise, then you have not been performing it correctly. Remember, intensity and force are both inversely proportional. As the level of exercise intensity and/or force increases during an exercise, then the length of time that exercise can be performed will proportionally decrease.

Initially, we also recommend that you perform only basic exercises for each body part. For example, you can perform either a power rack squat, wall squat, or an Iso-Bow® squat in 3 positions as isometric exercises. One position could be while your thighs are parallel to the floor, the next position about 20 degrees higher, and the last position about 20 degrees higher again. With those completed, you could then perform a Bullworker® squat, a power rack bar squat, or simply a freehand squat – all in super-slow exercise style.

Another example would be to perform a combination of an Iso-Bow®, Bullworker® or Steel Bow® chest press as an isometric exercise in three positions over the calculated range of motion. Then, after these have been completed, aim to perform 10 isotonic repetitions in super-slow exercise style using either the Bullworker®, or the Steel Bow, or by performing push-ups from either the toes or the knees. Once you have mastered achieving the 3 equal isometric exercise positions for each TRISOmetric™ exercise, then you have quite a wide selection of isotonic exercises to choose from to complete the exercise.

Super-Slow Training

I believe that it is almost impossible to move too slowly during an isotonic resistance exercise, however, it is easily possible to move too quickly. Super-slow is a form of strength training that was made popular by Ken Hutchins who worked at Nautilus and is based on an original concept by Dr Vincent Bocchicchio.

Dr Bocchicchio proposed that a single repetition of resistance training should take 10 seconds for the lifting phase, which is the concentric contraction where the muscles shorten. Then, pausing slightly to prevent momentum from being generated, after which it would take another 10 seconds to complete the lowering, or eccentric phase, where the muscles lengthen.

The super-slow concept incorporates extremely slow repetition speeds when compared to traditional resistance training protocols. In super-slow training, the emphasis is on minimizing momentum through minimal acceleration which, in turn, improves muscular loading. Most research suggests that super-slow training yields much better results in terms of strength gains and muscle growth than traditional resistance training methods.

The heart of the super-slow concept is based on the amount of tension a muscle develops. This is directly affected by the speed at which the muscle lengthens during the eccentric or lowering phase or shortens during the concentric or lifting phase of an exercise. The more tension that is generated, the more muscle fibres are recruited. More importantly, the slower the myosin and actin filaments within the muscle fibres slide past each other, the more links are formed between the filaments. Therefore, using super-slow exercise speeds a maximum amount of tension is generated and a higher number of filament links are formed. In short, super-slow training activates more muscle fibres at an increased rate to maintain the force necessary to move the resistance provided. This is why it is a very efficient way to increase both strength and muscle size.

A typical super-slow workout would consist of one set of each exercise which is performed to the point of complete muscle fatigue/failure. Therefore, a 10-repetition exercise in such a routine would take between 200 and 250 seconds to perform in practice, with the overall workout session taking no longer than 30 minutes to complete. Since this is a high-intensity system, it requires greater rest time between workout sessions. Therefore, a workout frequency of twice each week is typically recommended to avoid overtraining and burnout.

One of the great advantages of super-slow training is injury prevention. This is because in traditional resistance training, to make it more challenging more weight is added to increase the resistance used. Therefore, in and of itself, the traditional method naturally increases the risk of injury. However, with super-slow training, to make the exercise more challenging and engage more muscle fibres, simply slow the exercise down even more without there being a need to increase the weight.

A by-product of super-slow training is that it also produces some excellent cardiovascular benefits. This is because the heart is an involuntary muscle, therefore, it will always pump harder when there is more blood that needs pumping. Several studies have shown that super-slow training returns more blood to the heart than traditional aerobic training methods.

Strength at Only One Angle?

I have written quite a lot about dividing the ROM or Range of Motion of a limb roughly equally into three positions and then performing an isometric exercise at each point. Therefore, I thought I would make this clearer in pictures. Also, to explain away a common myth that isometric contraction exercises will only increase muscle strength at the specific angle at which the muscle and joint are exercised. When talking about building strength in a broader range, rather than at a more specific point, one of the first things that should also be remembered is that during regular isotonic weight training, a constant-curve range of strength gain is not achieved anyway. The data clearly shows that with respect to isometric exercise, it is only partially true that there is only an increase in strength at the angle the contraction is engaged. The scientific study performed by scientists Kitai and Sale called: "Specificity of Joint Angle in Isometric Training," concluded that strength gains were the greatest at the specific angle the training was performed. It also concluded that there was a significant increase in strength along a much wider strength curve than previously thought. The study showed that there were increases in strength at the angles of +5 degrees and -5 degrees to the isometric hold position.

More extensive studies have subsequently found that with isometric contraction exercises, there is often an even wider strength curve benefit than was first thought. The later studies found that between 20% and 50% of strength transfer occurs at the angles of +20 degrees, and -20 degrees to the isometric hold position. This is huge, and it completely dispels all myths about any potential issues about this. The additional research also concluded that for those athletes who wanted to achieve the most complete and constant curve strength gain, it was comparatively easy to achieve with isometric contraction exercises, especially when compared to regular isotonic weight training. In practical terms, to achieve the most complete and constant-curve strength gain possible, an advanced athlete would simply perform an isometric contraction exercise at two, three, or many more positions along the ROM of the body part being exercised. A normal, healthy limb has a certain Range of Motion, AKA: ROM. This is the arc through which the movement takes place at a joint, or series of joints. This ROM is technically called "Osteokinematic" motion.   Taking the biceps curl as an example, the range of motion for that movement in the pictures starts at zero when the hand is in the lower position and goes up to approximately 130 degrees in the upper position.

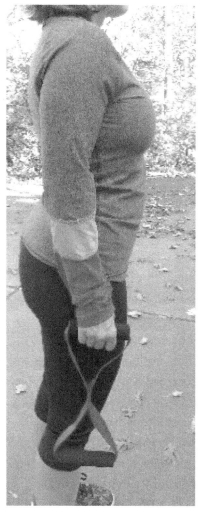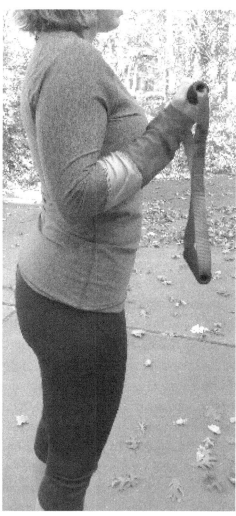

Zero Degrees   130 Degrees

Assuming that there is a strength-curve benefit of +20 degrees and -20 degrees around the point at which an isometric contraction is performed, then the first position would be at approximately 20 degrees from the neutral starting point because this would give a strength-curve benefit covering the first 40 degrees of the ROM.

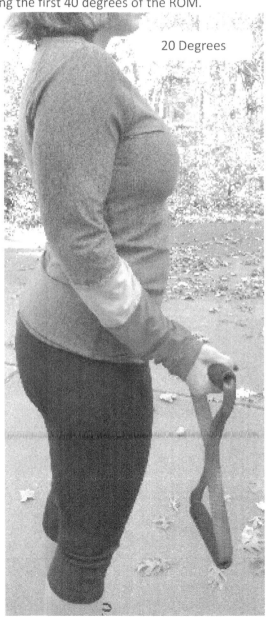

20 Degrees

The second position would be at approximately 50 degrees from the starting point which would safely overlap the first strength-curve arc from about the 30-degree point and extend up to about 70 degrees.

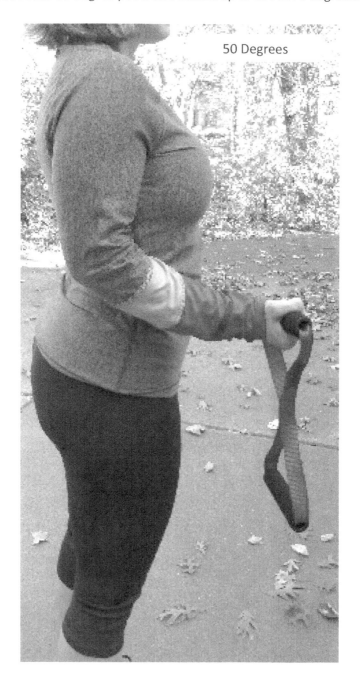

50 Degrees

The final position is at approximately 80 to 95 degrees from the starting point, overlapping the last point to provide a strength-curve benefit at the high end of the arc at circa 130 degrees of the maximum ROM.

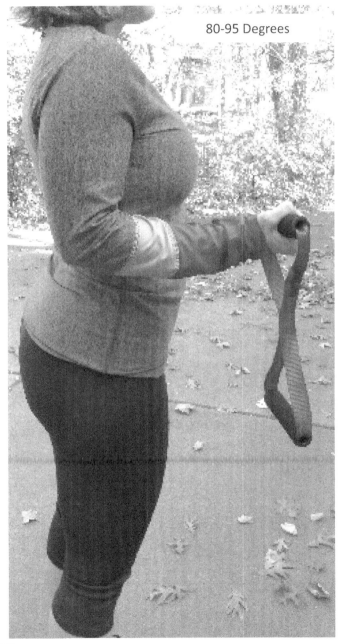

80-95 Degrees

If necessary, a highly advanced athlete might also want to add an isometric contraction exercise at both the starting and end position of the ROM. This would then strengthen the muscles when in the most mechanically disadvantaged position.

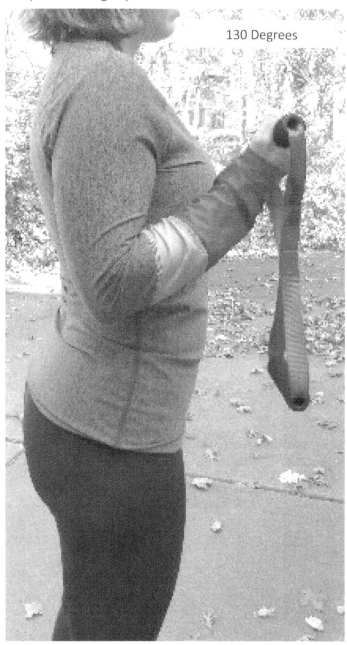

130 Degrees

Chapter 5: The Iso-Bow®

A common question we are asked is: "Is it necessary to use the Iso-Bow® to perform an effective isometric or self-resisted workout?" This is a good question. No, it is not necessary to use an Iso-Bow®, but we believe that it is better if you do, and there are several reasons why.

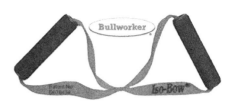

Firstly, it is all about the science and safety of biomechanics. A stable line of biomechanical progression all begins with a correctly positioned grip, a firm grip, and the progression in continuing that stability

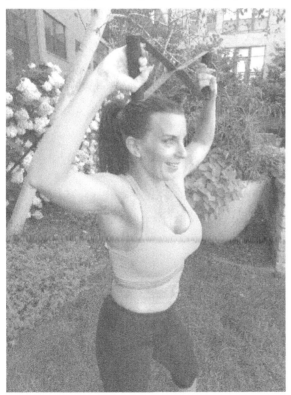

through correctly aligned joints and limbs while you perform the exercise. The same is true in isometric exercise because it all begins with a stable line of biomechanical progression. This starts with either a properly clenched hand or fist and continues that stability through correctly aligned joints and limbs to perform the isometric hold.

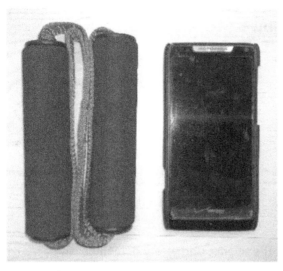

This is just one reason why we fully recommend and endorse the Iso-Bow® because it makes this whole process much easier. It has a well-designed and comfortable non-slip handgrip, which allows you to execute a firm, stable handgrip position to begin creating a stable line of biomechanical progression.

The Iso-Bow® is a product we fully endorse and highly recommend. It is inexpensive, and high quality, and most importantly, it works exceptionally well. An amazing Iso-Bow® costs "pennies" in comparison to other exercise devices, and even a pair of them can easily fit into your pocket, they never need adjusting, and they can deliver a total-body workout at the perfect level of intensity for either a completely unfit beginner or an advanced athlete!

If you have already read "The 70 Second Difference™" book, then you will also know that we are not even endorsing our product. We are simply endorsing a product that we believe will be the best investment you will ever make if you want to get fit, strong, and in

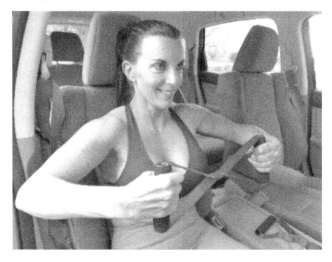

the best shape of your life. The company that makes the Iso-Bow® is Hughes Marketing LLC, and they also produce a small range of other highly effective exercise products, which all deliver excellent results at a fair price.

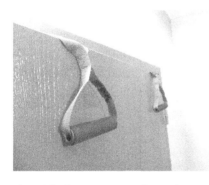

The Iso-Bow® is versatile too, and it can be used with equal effectiveness as both an isotonic and an isometric exercise device. It allows the user to perform highly effective self-resisted isotonic exercises for almost every muscle group.

A pair of Iso-Bows® can even be used as a great doorway pull-up device, which can even fold up and

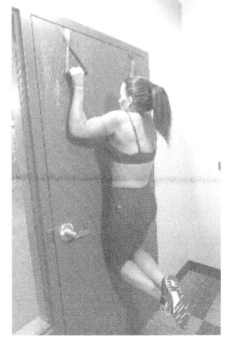

slip right into your pocket when you are done. Try doing that with a regular, clumsy steel doorway pull-up bar!

The Iso-Bow® is naturally a first-class isometric exercise device, and it allows a very wide range of exercises to be performed that work almost every muscle group of the body. It also allows the effective execution of more advanced techniques to be performed within the ISOfitness™ system.

Since the Iso-Bow® is inexpensive, well-designed, well-constructed, and extremely useful in ways we have not even begun to describe here in this book, it is not so much a recommendation for you to get a pair, but rather an instruction for you to do so. We believe that you will soon see why these inexpensive devices are what we believe to be the finest, most versatile, and most powerful of all exercise devices that have ever been invented!

That is a bold statement, but it is made because of our sincere belief in the product, and how you will benefit from owning a pair if you use them correctly. Do not forget, that we do not make this product, we simply believe in it to that degree of commitment.

Securing the Iso-Bow® With Your Feet

When performing leg exercises such as squats and lunges, as well as lower back and glute exercises such as the deadlift, it becomes necessary to properly secure the Iso-Bow® using your feet.

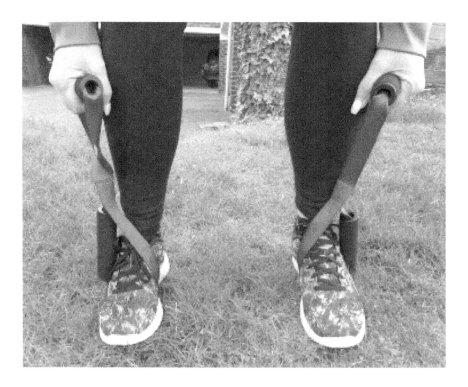

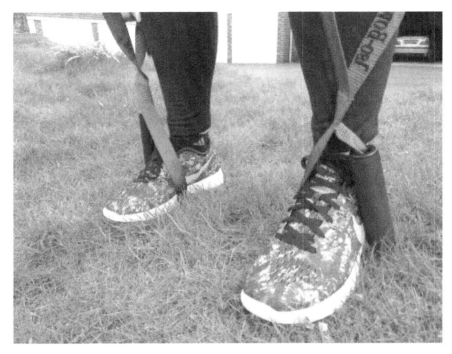

There are several ways in which the Iso-Bow® can be secured using your feet, and your personal preference of how you do this will depend upon many factors such as your foot size, your choice of footwear, and ease of operation. You can secure the Iso-Bow® with your foot inside one of the handles. You do this by adjusting the handgrip to one side, usually the outer side of the foot, and then placing your feet inside the loop like a stirrup.

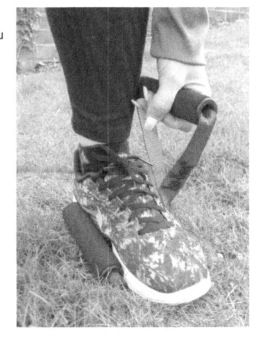

Another method is to place the Iso-Bow® flat on the

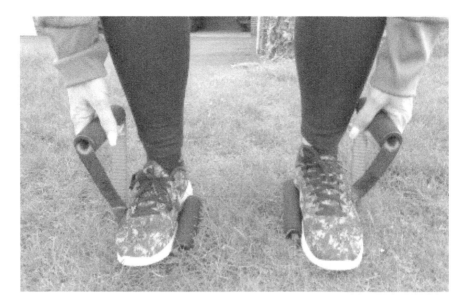

floor and then stand on one side of the straps so that the handle of the same side sits flush with your inner foot. In this position, it will be your bodyweight combined with the handle pressing against the inner side of your foot which enables you to pull safely and securely.

The final method is to simply place each foot through one end of an Iso-Bow®, stepping onto the foam handgrip as you do so. This method is slightly less stable than the other two methods. However, if the foot can be pushed far enough through the loop of the Iso-Bow® handle, then the handle will slightly

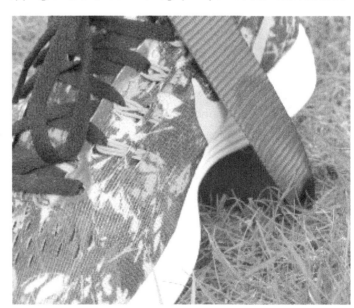

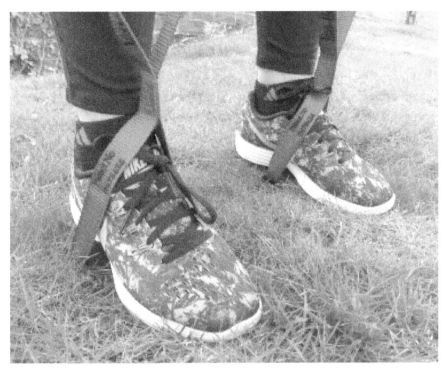

raise the level of your heel making it easier for some people to squat or lunge. Naturally, safety is always a top priority so whichever method you ultimately choose to use, you should always make sure that when securing the Iso-Bow® with your feet there is never any chance of it slipping in any way while you exercise.

Shortening The Iso-Bow® - The Cradle

Generally, the Iso-Bow® is the ideal size for most people to use with each exercise. However, occasionally you may prefer to reduce its operational size by roughly half, by creating what we call an Iso-Bow® cradle.

To do this you place one of the handles inside the webbing loop of the other handle side of the device. The handle you have just placed inside the loop is then cradled by the webbing and can be gripped as normal. Your thumb and fingers can then wrap around both the foam handle and the webbing of the cradle loop to help ensure an even firmer grip position is created.

This reduced size allows for an even greater operational range within the movement capability of each limb/joint to be created for certain exercises. These include The Cross-Chest Press, the Upper Back Power Pull, and the Biceps and Triceps Cradle Press-Curl.

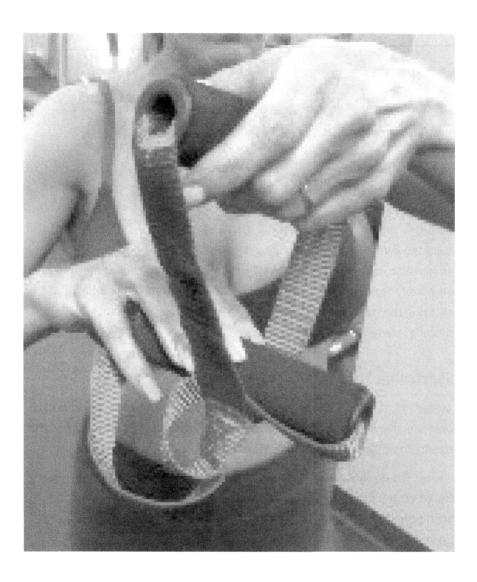

Proprietary and Readily Available Equipment

The Bullworker® Classic

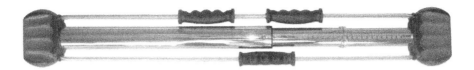

The Bullworker® Classic is approximately 36 inches long and can be used either as a stand-alone device or as a complete home gym when in combination with the Steel Bow® and the Iso-Bow®. It currently has several interchangeable springs with different levels of resistance. More may be added in the future to allow an even greater range of people to use the device for an even wider range of exercises. Today, with the shift towards more people choosing to exercise at home, the Bullworker has *now become the total-body all-in-one compact personal gym of choice.*

The Steel Bow®

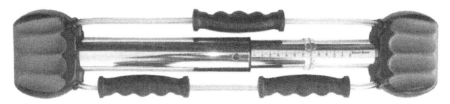

The Steel Bow® is about 20 inches long and is simply a shorter version of the full-size Bullworker® Classic model and comes with several interchangeable springs of varying levels of resistance.

IIEDs or Improvised Isometric Exercise Devices

One of the best things about isometric exercises is that if you do not want to use traditional gym equipment or proprietary devices, then you do not have to use them to perform a full workout. Instead, you can either use nothing at all except your own body, immovable objects such as doors, walls, and door jambs, or readily available everyday items.

These can include walking sticks/poles, broom handles, towels, and a sturdy towing or climbing rope. I will outline some of these items as suggestions for alternative equipment/devices you can use for your workout sessions.

The Walking Stick/Pole

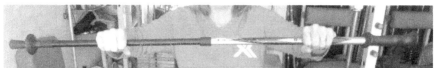

The walking stick or pro-style walking pole is an excellent device to use for an isometric workout. It is the equivalent of a barbell or Bullworker® Classic without the steel cables at each side. One of the great advantages the pro-style walking pole offers is that it can be adjusted to various lengths, which makes it easily adaptable for use in a variety of exercises. Many of the exercises can be performed alone, without any need for partner assistance. An even greater range of exercises can be performed if a workout partner is available. Nordic Walking Poles are slightly different from ordinary walking poles, but they work equally well for isometric exercises.

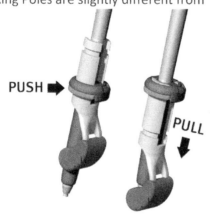

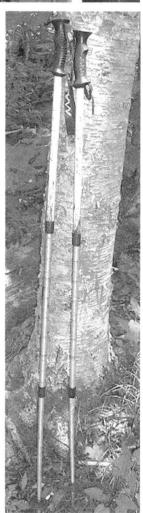

Nordic Walking Pole Tip by: Tslmarketing

Photo: Daniel Case

The Humble Beach or Bath Towel

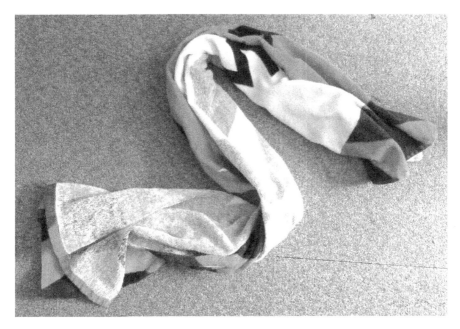

The humble beach or bath towel is a common tool used by isometric enthusiasts who have nothing else to exercise with. It is also an exercise tool of choice for many because it is incredibly versatile.

When choosing a towel to exercise with, the important things to look for are that it must be long enough, it must also be flexible enough to enable you to grip it properly, and therefore, it must not be too thick. Naturally, it must also be in good condition and not be liable to tear or rip during your exercise session.

Rope – Either Climbing Rope or Towing Rope

A rope is another remarkably simple but highly effective tool that can be used to perform an isometric and/or self-resisted workout routine. the important things to look for in a rope that might be suitable for exercise use are, sufficient length, it must be thick enough to allow a comfortable handgrip, and it must be in good condition so that it will not break during your workout routine.

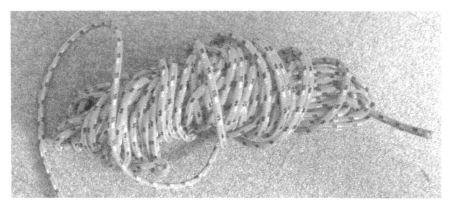

If you are using your feet to secure the rope, then for added safety and comfort you may wish to loop the rope around the foot as shown. This will make it less likely to slip when it is pulled hard, and it will be more comfortable for the foot as well.

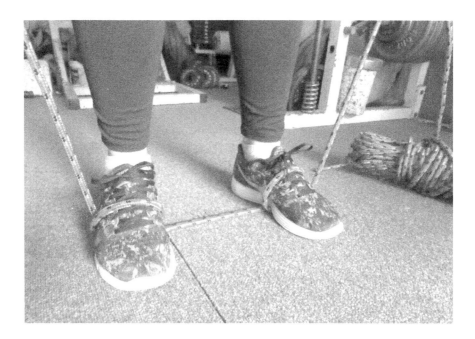

The Broom Handle

The broom handle can be used almost identically to the walking stick or pro-style walking pole. By its very nature, it is not nearly as flexible as a walking stick or pro-style walking pole.

This is because you can easily take a walking stick or pro-style walking pole virtually anywhere. After all, that is precisely what they have been designed for.

You would appear to be very odd indeed if you were to carry around a broom with you to exercise with, whereas a walking stick or pro-style walking pole would not look even the slightest bit out of place.

If you use a broom handle at home to exercise with, then make sure it is solid and will not break when used in a workout routine.

Also, we would strongly caution against using one to support your body weight in any way with the broom handle to support it.

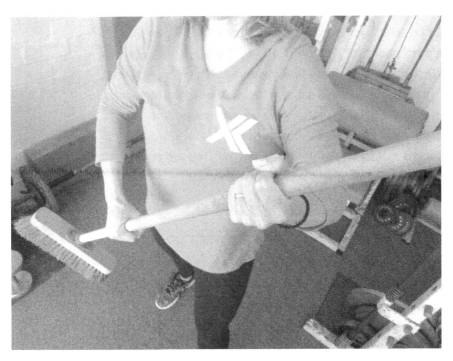

The Climber's Sling

The climber's sling, or any kind of climbing-grade webbing/material for that matter, almost always makes an ideal IIED or Improvised Isometric Exercise Device. A climbing sling, or runner, is an item of basic equipment climbers use. It is either a tied or sewn loop of webbing that can be attached to a carabiner or around a rock and hitched (tied) to other equipment. Climber's slings are extremely useful because the longer ones can be easily double-looped, or more, to reduce their circumference by half with every reducing loop added. This makes the longer slings an extremely versatile IIED because the length and thickness can be easily and quickly adjusted according to the isometric exercise you wish to perform.

Professionally sewn and bonded climber's slings are extremely strong with a typical average breaking strength of at least 22 kilonewtons or 4,900 lbf. To give you a better frame of reference to the breaking strain of a 22 kN climbing sling, an average Range Rover Sport SUV weighs about 4,727 lb or 2,144 kg. Therefore, a typical 22 kN climbing sling made from nylon webbing is more than capable of being used safely as an IIED, or any other kind of exercise for that matter. When undamaged and properly made, they cannot be ripped apart during exercise, or by any other form of human muscle power, not even by The World's Strongest Man.

The Climber's Daisy Chain

Another excellent and versatile IIED or Improvised Isometric Exercise Device found in the typical range of equipment sold in a climbing store is the daisy chain.

A daisy chain is a webbing chain strap that is several feet/centimetres long. Typically, it is made from approximately one-inch (2.54 cm) nylon webbing of the same or similar type to that used in climbing slings and lengthening straps between anchor points and the main climbing rope.

The webbing is securely stitched at intervals of approximately two inches to form loops on one side along the length of the main webbing strap.

Alternatively, and these are the type we prefer, the nylon webbing is sewn into a series of closely spaced interlocked loops to create a looped daisy chain for the desired length of the device.

At one end there is usually a much larger foot loop to accommodate a climbing boot, and at the other end, there is a carabiner point made from a smaller piece of nylon webbing in a tight loop or bite.

A Typical Climber's Daisy Chain

Note the Foot Loop at One End and the Carabiner Point/s at the Other End

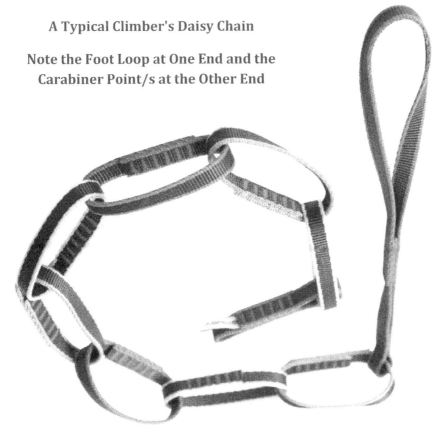

Conclusion

Since the isometric exercise requires no limb movement, it is very easy to perform a wide range of effective exercises using the self-resistance method.

Therefore, one can use just about any device that is unbreakable by human muscle power alone. However, as with all things, using a proprietary device that is purpose-made will always make it easier, and sometimes safer to perform.

One of the good things about all of the example devices shown in this section is that none could be considered to be expensive, and all are built to a high standard of quality and durability. In short, the choice is yours and whatever you choose will deliver good results!

Chapter 6: About the Exercise Model

Unless you have skipped the entire first part of this book, you will already know a great deal about me. However, for those who have skipped that section to get right down to the exercises, here is a brief recap and gallery showing what I achieved with the minimum of time spent exercising.

Helen Renée is an American who is married to a Brit. She was born in Minnesota and grew up in Northern Alaska after her father became an Ice Road Trucker. She went from being 40-50 lbs overweight to a contest-winning condition almost effortlessly in less than 6 months and with workout sessions lasting no longer than 10 minutes per day.

Helen is an isometric exercise expert instructor and champion Bikini Fitness Athlete who achieved spectacular contest-winning results after meeting her exercise scientist husband. Helen's husband is one of the world's leading experts on isometric exercise, plant-based nutrition, and was a former coach to the 4-times World's Strongest Man, Jon Pall Sigmarsson of Iceland. Currently, Helen has co-authored 22 fitness books and since she and her husband share a common fascination with mysteries and the paranormal, they have co-authored a best-selling book on the subject. Helen is remarkably strong with the exceptional power-to-weight ratio one would expect from a former gymnast. She is also an isometric and TRISOmetric™ exercise instructor, consultant, and instructor-trainer for TWiEA™ The World Isometric Exercise Association. www.TWiEA.com – www.HelenRenee.com

Since meeting and marrying her British husband, they have enjoyed a joyous journey together discovering the many differences between the two countries which share a common language and culture. They began writing these stories and anecdotes down and very soon had enough to produce a fun-filled and light-hearted book about what it is like Being American Married to a Brit.

The following pictures are of Helen Renée taken in January 2015 before she started performing a daily 10 x 7-second total-body exercise isometric exercise routine.

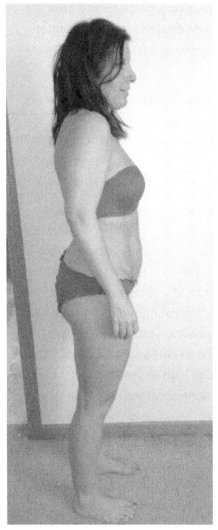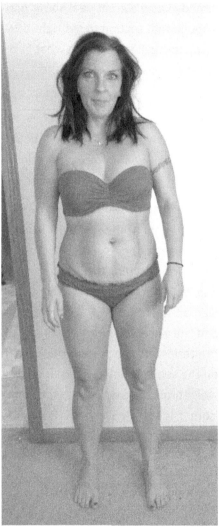

The following pictures are of Helen Renée 1-year later, in January 2016. She became a contest-winning Bikini Fitness competitor within 1-year of daily isometric exercise training lasting only minutes each day. Now, Helen trains using only isometric exercises because they are so effective and time-saving. She simply exercises regularly each day and applies more force to each exercise than a normal person who simply wants to get a little stronger, fitter, and maintain a good overall body shape. Helen also eats sensibly.

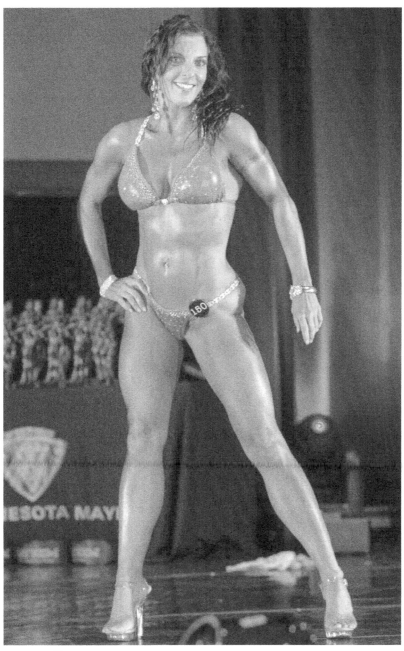

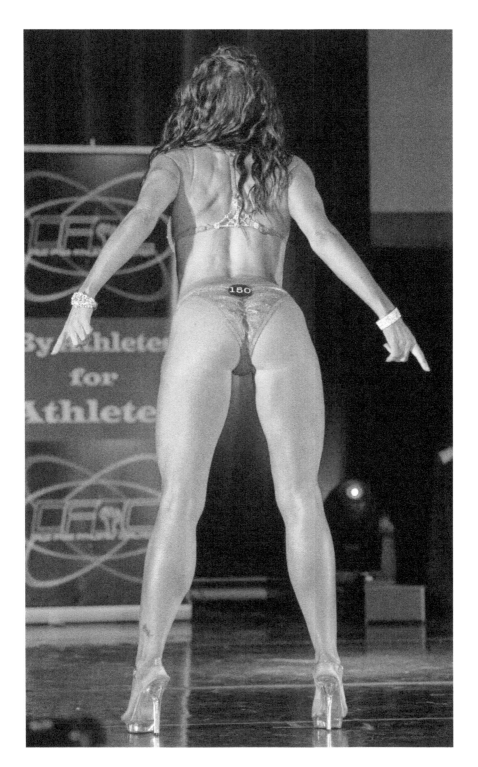

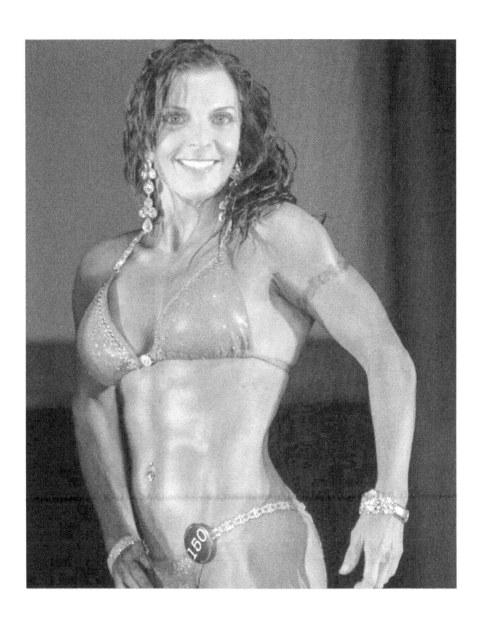

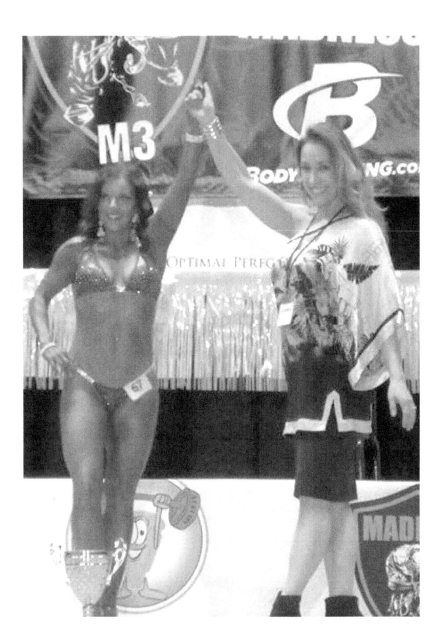

The Authors and an Isometric Experiment

I am Brian, Helen's co-author, and the following picture is of my arm taken in December 2016. This was after a year-long experiment to see what results could be gained through a basic high-intensity isometric exercise routine using only the minimum number of exercises.

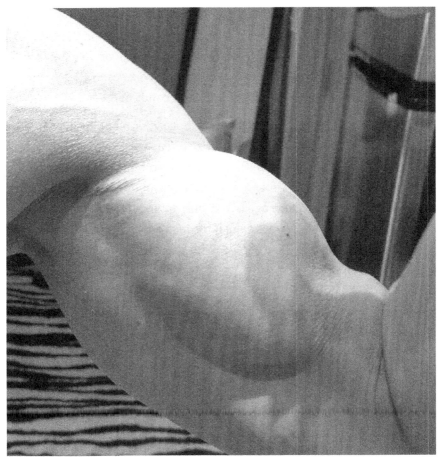

My arm after 1 year of basic isometric maintenance training.
This picture was taken to record the results of the experiment in December 2016.
The experimental training routine allowed just 1 x 7-second isometric exercise per muscle/muscle group per day at a target level of applied force/intensity of between 75% and 80% of my estimated maximum.

For one year, starting in January 2016, I performed a daily 10-exercise x 7-second total-body isometric routine. It is common for even the most experienced athletes to count the elapsed exercise time increasingly quickly, almost in direct proportion to an increasing level of applied force/intensity. Therefore, I typically aimed to perform a 10-second isometric hold for each exercise, and this way I would always reach the desired goal of 7 seconds in good style.

My target level of force for each exercise was around 75-80%, slightly higher than the typically recommended average of only 2/3^{rds}, or 66.6%. However, this still effectively meant that I exercised each of my biceps for a total of between just 21 and 30 seconds per week.

Amazingly, at the end of the year-long experiment, I achieved an improvement in both the strength and size of each arm, albeit slight. Even though I am well-versed in the science of isometrics I still found it remarkable because it was in exchange for a maximum of 30 seconds per week of exercise time. Once again, this only served to reinforce the fact that the best results are always gained through pinpoint focus, high intensity, and never confusing activity with accomplishment.

Chapter 7:
Things to Remember and Tips Before You Begin

▲ The first and perhaps the most important thing to remember is: **NEVER HOLD YOUR BREATH AT ANY TIME.**

▲ Breathing in and out naturally during all isometric exercises will also help you count the number of elapsed seconds much more accurately, with one full breath in and out taking approximately one second.

▲ We recommend that you read the instructions about each exercise carefully. You can also watch the associated videos via the TWiEA™ website if you wish to become a member and access those resources.

▲ Always leave a safe distance between you and others if exercising with any proprietary device or IIED (Improvised Isometric Exercise Device)

▲ Always check the structural integrity of any type of exercise device. If there is any doubt about the structural integrity, then do not use it for exercise or any other purpose.

▲ Double-check that any/all adjustable joints on the exercise device and/or IIED are secure before use.

▲ Weight loss/fat loss will ONLY occur when any exercise plan is used in conjunction with a calorie-controlled diet.

▲ It is critically important to completely focus your mind on the exercise being performed. Envision the muscle you are exercising as growing larger and stronger.

▲ Always consult a professional coach to devise a detailed stretching routine, this will ensure that you are stretching the areas effectively rather than risking injury.

▲ Always ensure that a stable line of biomechanical progression is achieved before engaging in and performing any exercise.

◭ Warming-up, stretching, and cooling down are three of the most overlooked yet essential elements of exercise, and we cannot stress their importance strongly enough.

◭ During ANY form of physical exercise, including isometrics, if you apply too much force too soon, then you may inadvertently strain a muscle. Isometric exercise can be intense, and a single isometric exercise engages a great many more muscle fibres than even high-intensity weight training does, and at a much higher level too.

For safety's sake, we recommend using Dynamic Flexation™ to engage your muscles gradually and progressively into ANY exercise according to our ISOfitness Exercise Engagement Timeline™.

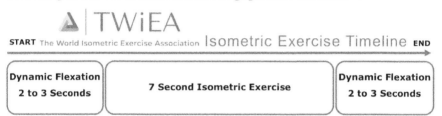

The main benefit of properly warming-up for several minutes before a workout is injury prevention and increasing your heart rate and circulation to your muscles, ligaments, and tendons. In addition to properly warming-up, always perform a gentle flex and stretch of the muscles and joints which are about to be exercised. For example, squatting down fully to flex the thighs and loosen the knees is always a good idea before performing any leg exercises.

Dynamic Flexation™ performed before any exercise should help to ensure greater flexibility and increased blood supply to the muscles and surrounding tissue. It is important to remember that warming-up and stretching are two different concepts and that stretching is not a good warm-up. This is because stretching will put the muscle in an uncontracted position and weaken it. Stretching is always best performed after a workout has been completed, together with a proper cool-down regimen.

Charts of the Major Muscle Groups

The following charts showing the major muscle groups should help you to better identify the ones you are targeting in each exercise. The better acquainted you become with the muscle groups and their basic function, the better your exercise style should become.

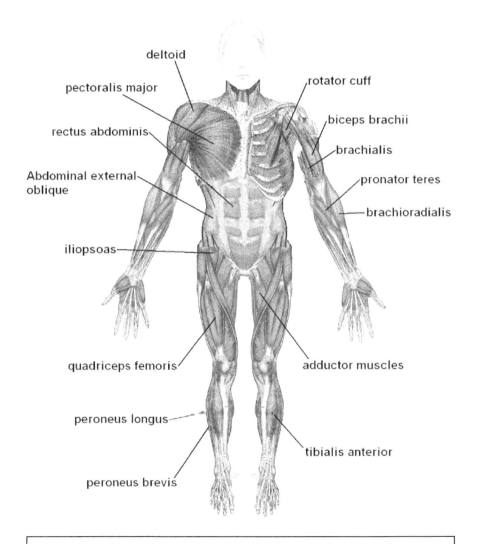

deltoid

pectoralis major

rectus abdominis

Abdominal external oblique

iliopsoas

quadriceps femoris

peroneus longus

peroneus brevis

rotator cuff

biceps brachii

brachialis

pronator teres

brachioradialis

adductor muscles

tibialis anterior

> **Frontal (anterior) View of the Main Human Skeletal Muscles**

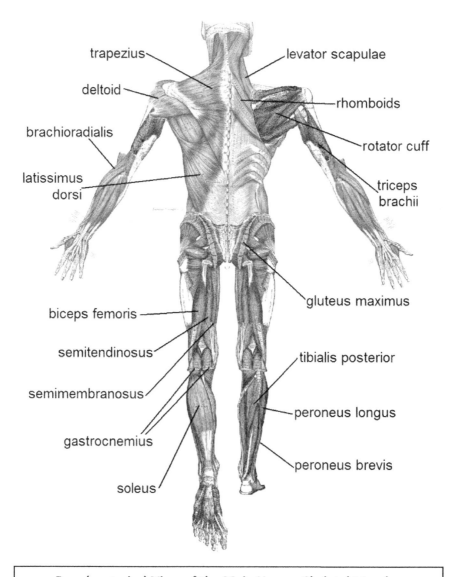

Rear (posterior) View of the Main Human Skeletal Muscles

Isometric exercises are deceptively powerful. Even when engaging in what may feel like only moderate-intensity exercise, you are probably still engaging and contracting many more muscle fibres than you would in a similar isotonic exercise. Therefore, if you are in any doubt whatsoever, then always perform the exercise with a little less intensity.

All exercises and workout plans work equally well for men and women. Both sexes can build strength, muscle, body build, or simply get into great shape if so desired, each according to their natural ability.

In our exercise resource books, the exercises listed are suggestions of what can be performed for each body part/muscle group. We are not suggesting that they should all be performed. Instead, users may wish to select the most suitable exercises from each section. In our course books, please perform the exercises according to the workout session notes.

Finally, please read, review, and ensure that you have fully complied with all recommendations in the section headed, Important General Safety and Health Guidelines.

Finally, only start using the isometric, or any other exercise system with the full approval of your physician.

Chapter 8: The Workout at Work™ Workout

Abdominals: Knee Raise and Trunk Curl

Sit on a chair or any other solid object and place the Iso-Bow® with handles facing downwards, over the top of one knee.

Next, curl your body forwards and downwards by contracting the abdominals, and at the same time, raise the knee resisted by the Iso-Bow®. In doing so, press down on the knee to prevent it from rising too far.

Always breathe deeply and naturally as you perform the exercise, which will be about 10 full breaths, at a rate of about 1 second per breath.

Perform each exercise for no less than 7 seconds, and no longer than 10. Repeat the exercise using the other knee.

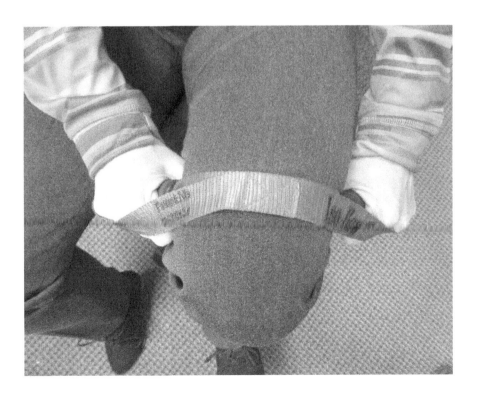

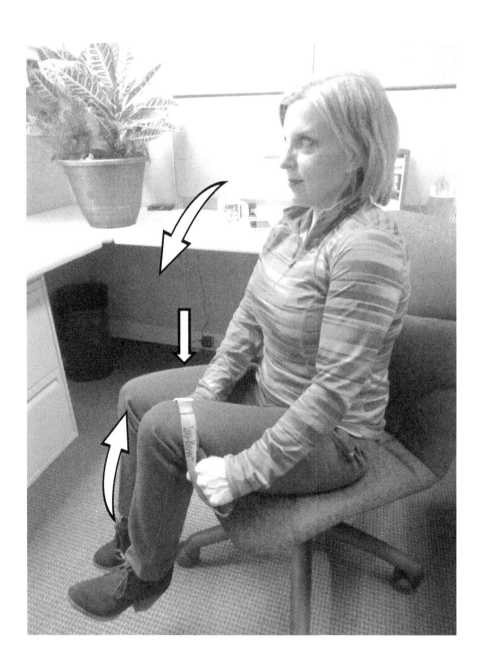

Alternative Method Without an Iso-Bow®

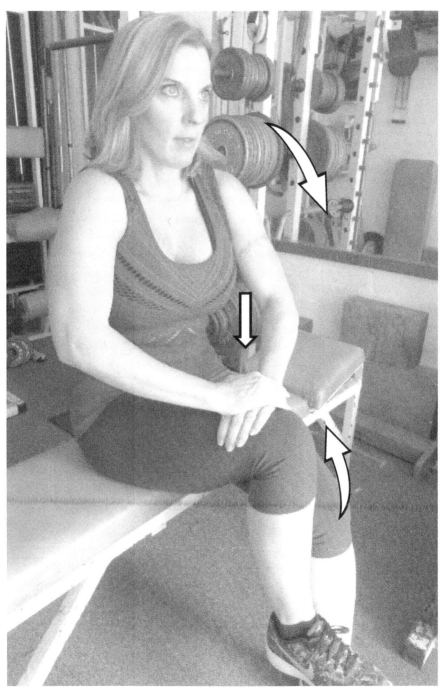

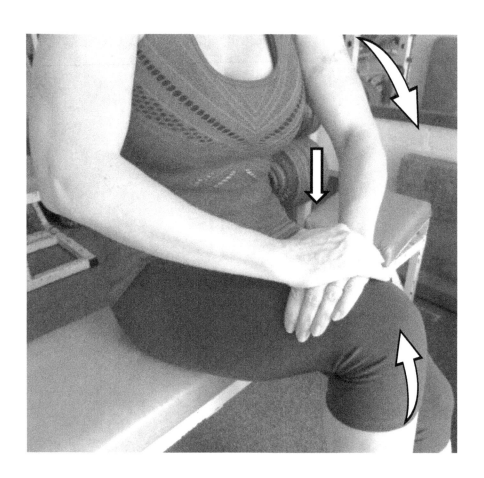

Arms: Biceps and Triceps

Iso-Bow® Biceps and Triceps Cradle Press-Curl (Left and Right Side)

Firstly, you need to learn how to make an Iso-Bow® cradle.

This is where you effectively reduce the size of the Iso-Bow® by half by placing one of the handles inside the webbing loop on the other side of the device.

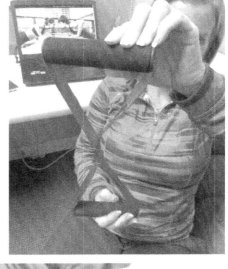

The handle you have just placed inside the loop is then cradled by the webbing and can be gripped as normal. Your thumb and

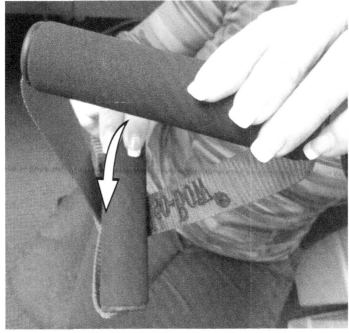

fingers can then wrap around both the foam handle and the webbing of the cradle-loop, to help ensure that a firm grip position is created.

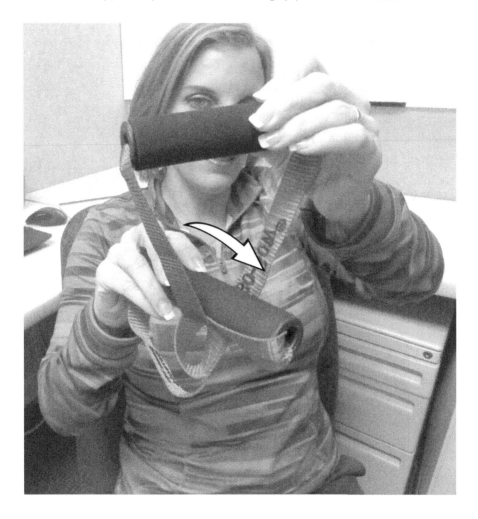

To perform the exercises, first, cradle the Iso-Bow® with your right hand, gripping the top and with your left hand facing upwards. Grip the cradled side of the Iso-Bow® with the right hand facing down. Keep both elbows close to your body, and with your left arm across the front of you at waist height.

In this position, press down with the right hand, and at the same time press up with the left. This will simultaneously engage the Biceps muscles on one arm, and the Triceps muscles on the other arm.

Breathe naturally and deeply, in and out, for about 10 full breaths, which will take about 1 second per breath. Aim to perform an exercise breathing count of no less than 7 seconds, and no longer than 10 seconds. Repeat the same exercise for the other arm by simply reversing the gripping process.

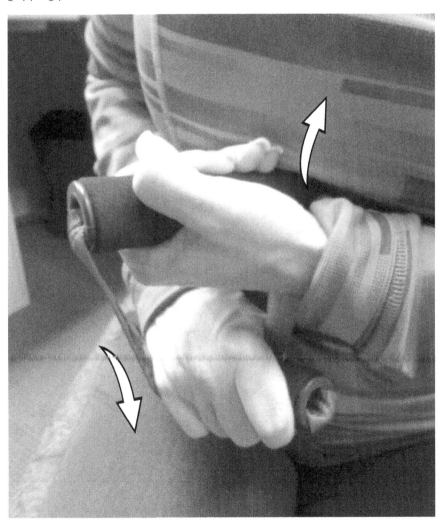

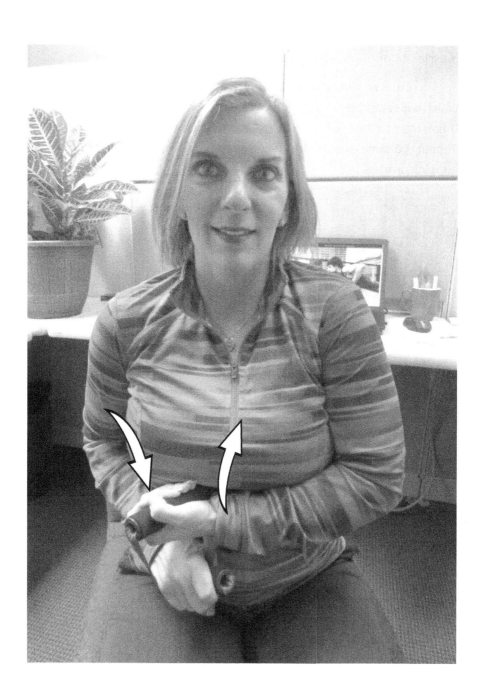

Repeat the same exercise by simply reversing the gripping process and hand position to the other side of the body to exercise other opposing muscle groups of the arms.

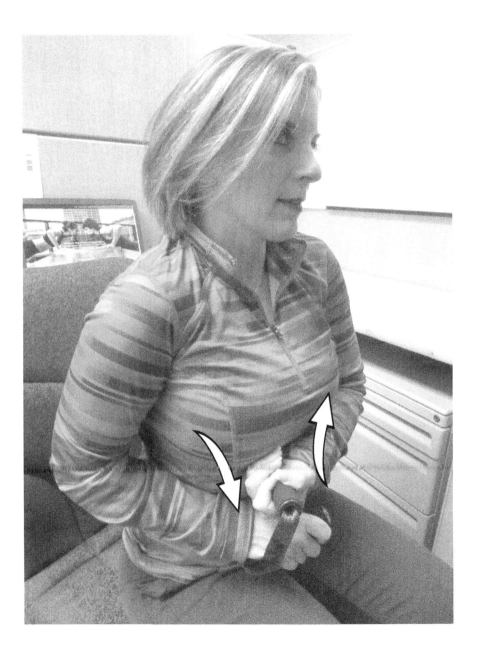

Alternative Biceps and Triceps Simultaneous Dual Exercises Without an Iso-Bow®

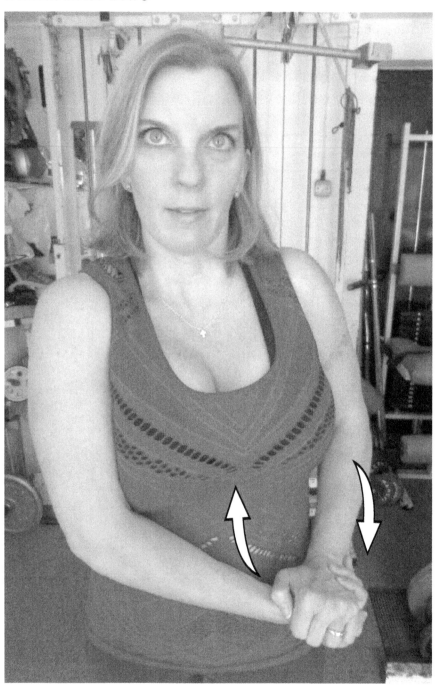

Do not forget to change sides & reverse the grip

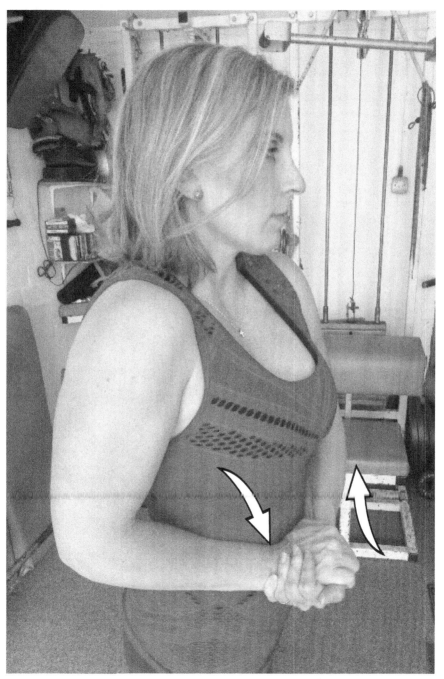

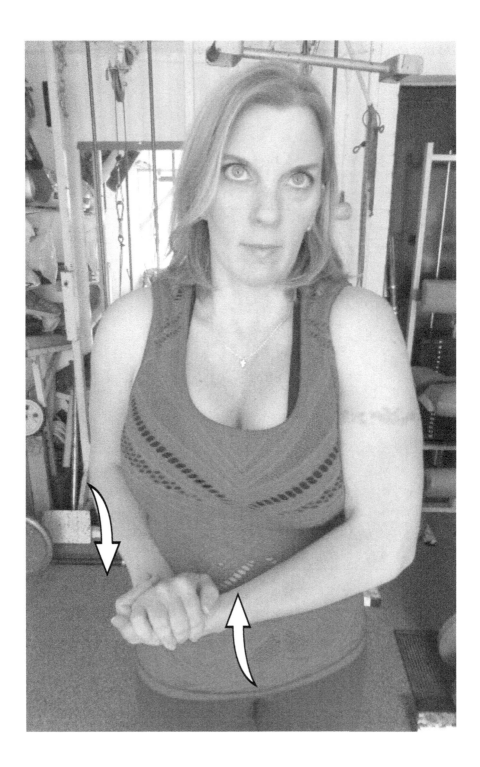

Dual Iso-Bow® Foot Loop Biceps Curl

Sit on a chair or any other solid object. Raise one leg and place the Iso-Bows® around each foot as shown.

In that position, pull up to engage the Biceps, while at the same time pushing the foot down to provide immovable resistance.

Breathe naturally and deeply in and out for about 10 full breaths, which will take about 1 second per breath.

Aim to perform an exercise breathing count of no less than 7 seconds, and no longer than 10 seconds.

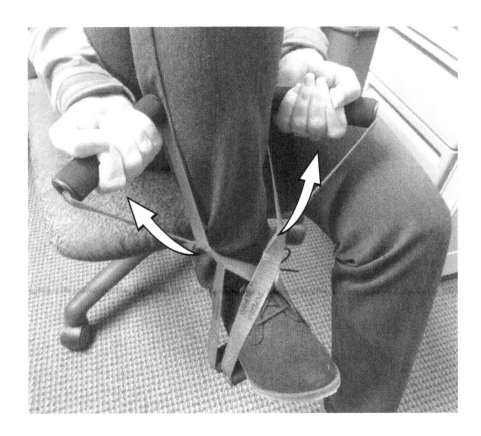

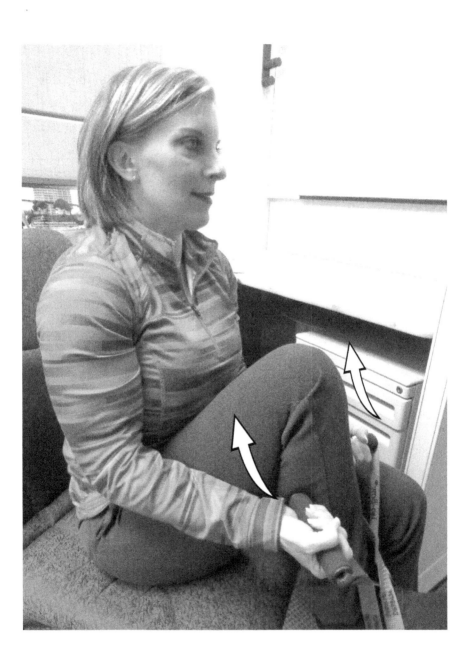

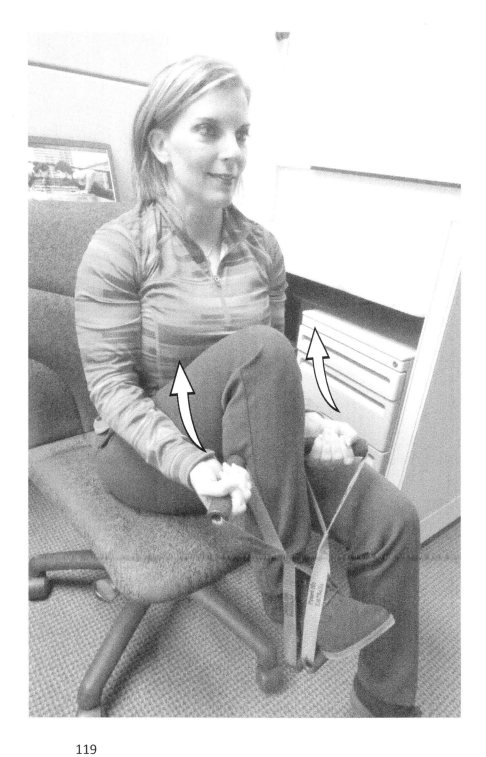

Iso-Bow® Shin-Resisted Biceps Curl

Sit on a chair or any other solid object. Raise one leg and place the Iso-Bow® comfortably just below the knee.

Pull up to engage the Biceps muscles of both arms, using the knee and leg to provide immovable resistance.

Breathe naturally and deeply in and out for about 10 full breaths, which will take about 1 second per breath.

Aim to perform an exercise breathing count of no less than 7 seconds, and no longer than 10 seconds.

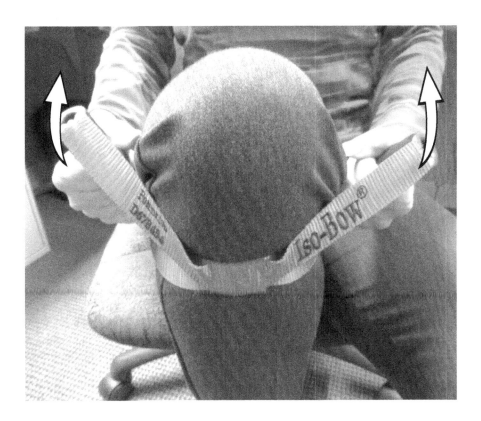

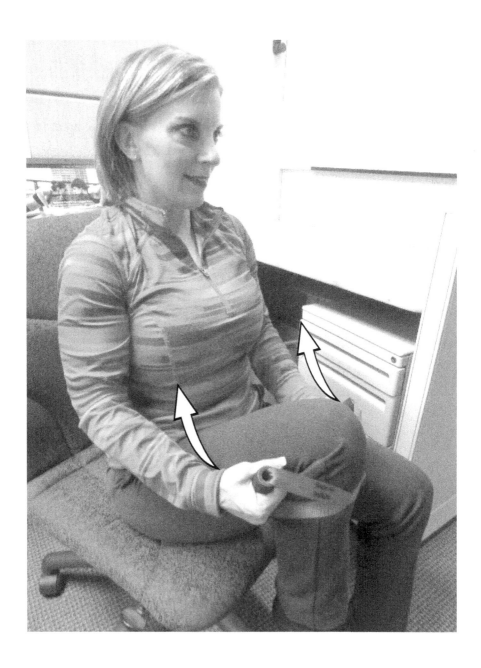

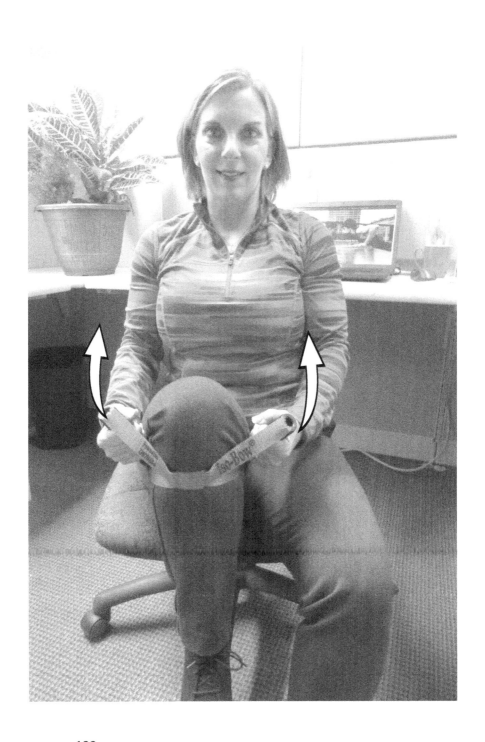

Iso-Bow® Triceps Front Press - Right and Left Arm

Hold the Iso-Bow® up to your shoulder and grip the handle firmly.

Hold the other handle with your hand facing away from you, keeping your arm and elbow at a 90-degree angle.

Engage the triceps muscles of the bent arm, by attempting to push your hand away against the resistance provided by your hand securing the Iso-Bow®.

Breathe naturally and deeply in and out for about 10 full breaths, which will take about 1 second per breath.

Aim to perform an exercise breathing count of no less than 7 seconds, and no longer than 10 seconds.

Repeat on the other side by reversing the action.

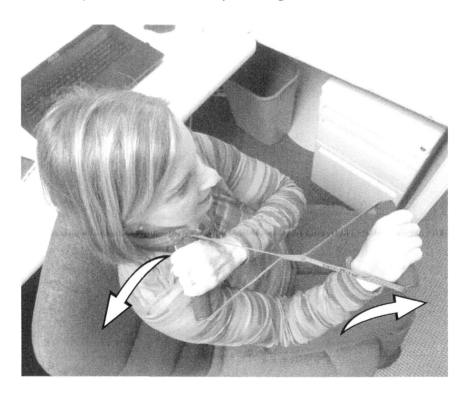

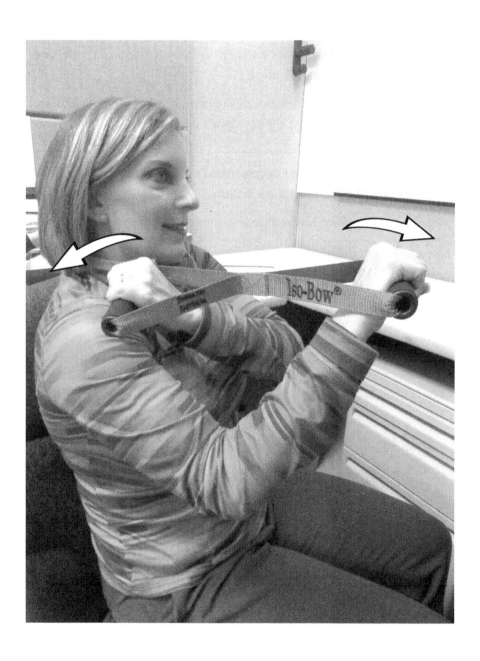

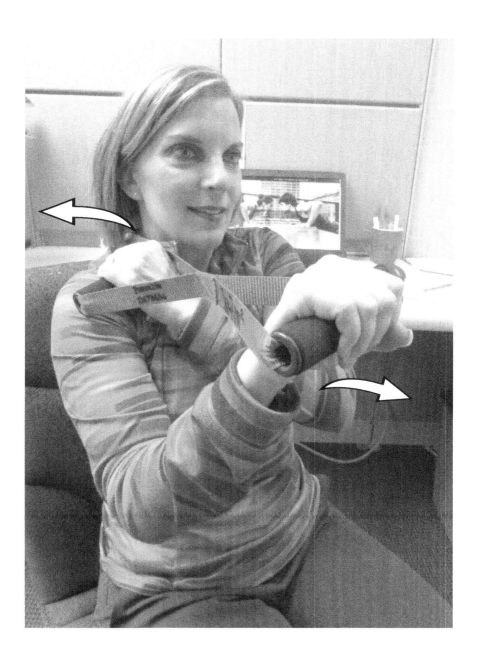

127
127

Forearms:

Iso-Bow® Seated Wrist Curl and Extension

Place an Iso-Bow® around each foot as shown and grip each handle with your palms facing down.

In this position, curl the gripping hand upwards to engage the extensor muscles of the upper forearm.

Breathe naturally and deeply in and out for about 10 full breaths, which will take about 1 second per breath.

Aim to perform an exercise breathing count of no less than 7 seconds, and no longer than 10 seconds.

Switch your grip so that your palms are facing up. Curl the gripping hand upwards to repeat the exercise for the flexor muscles of your inner forearm.

Palms Facing Down Grip

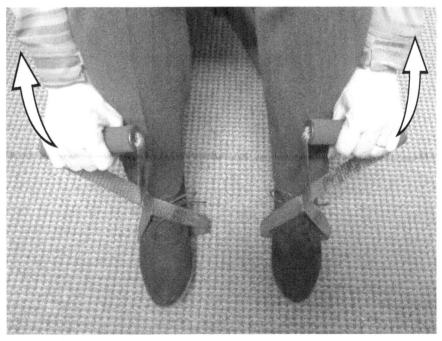

129

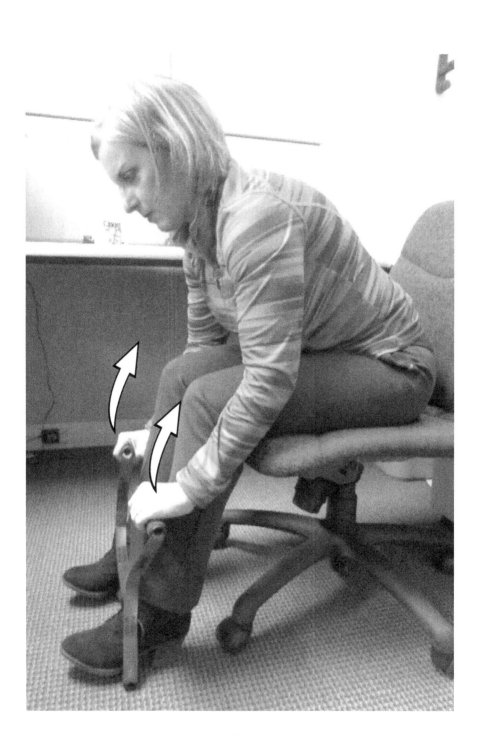

Palms Facing Up Grip

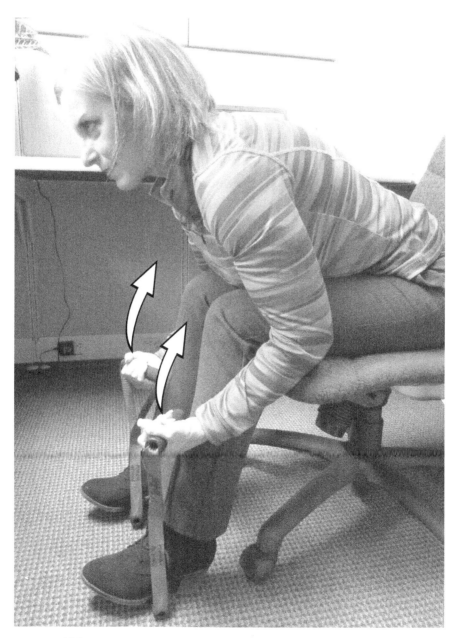

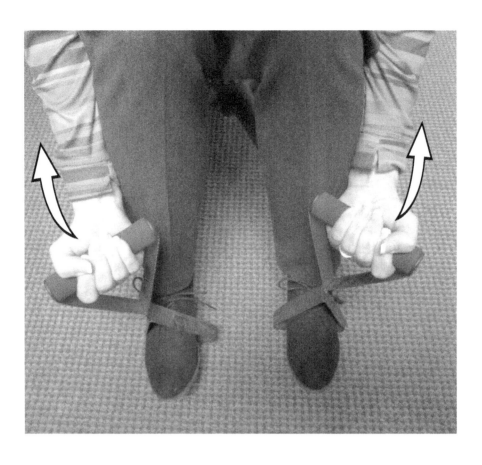

Alternative Exercise Without an Iso-Bow®

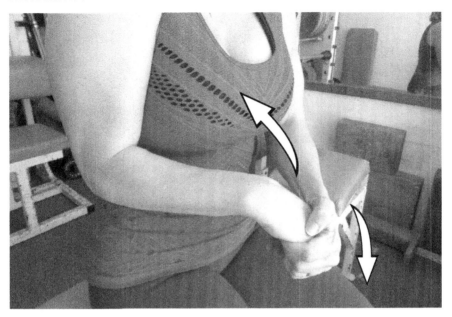

Reverse Hand Position

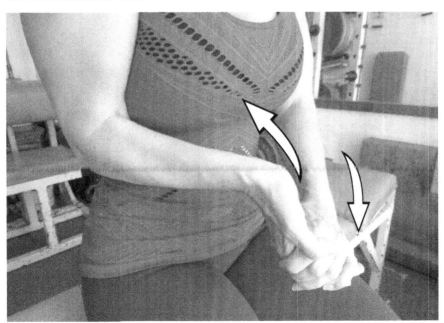

Back: Upper
Iso-Bow® Latissimus Overhead Pull Apart

Grip the Iso-Bow® handles with both hands and aim to position the central section comfortably, just above the top of the head.

In this position, try to pull your hands apart, engaging the latissimus muscles of the upper back as you do so.

Breathe naturally and deeply in and out for about 10 full breaths, which will take about 1 second per breath.

Aim to perform an exercise breathing count of no less than 7 seconds, and no longer than 10 seconds.

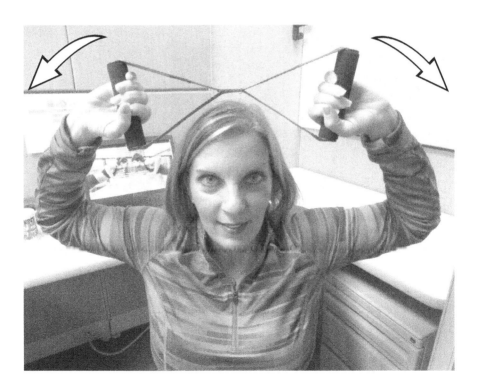

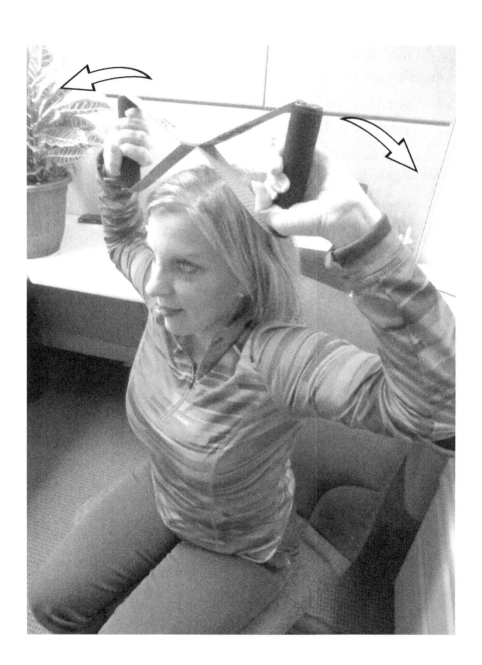

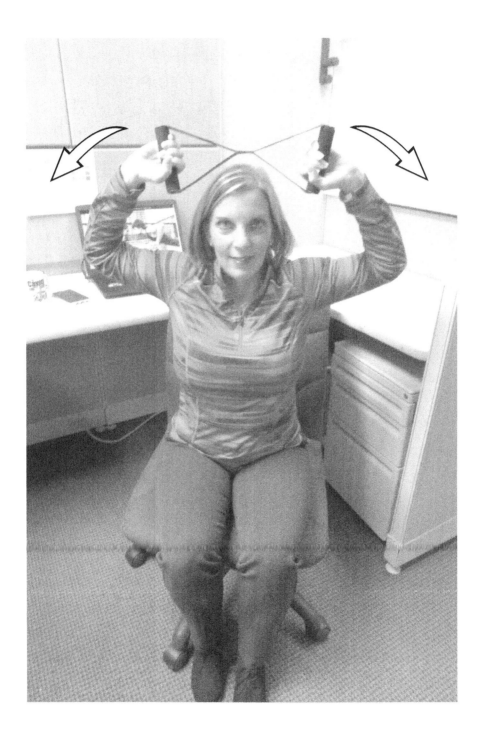

Alternative Exercise Without an Iso-Bow®

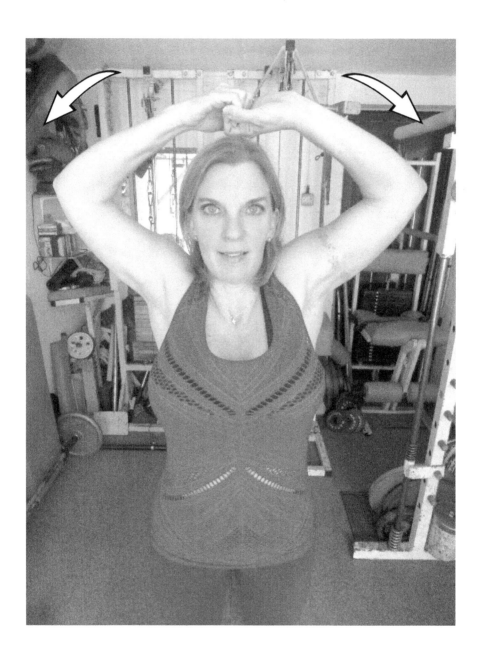

Iso-Bow® Back Power Cradle-Pull Mid and Wide

Firstly, cradle the Iso-Bow® to effectively half its size for a mid-width grip. Then, hold the Iso-Bow® in front of you, with your arms bent, and approximately parallel to the floor. In this position, attempt to pull the Iso-Bow® apart to engage the central upper back muscles.

Breathe naturally and deeply in and out for about 10 full breaths, which will take about 1 second per breath.   Aim to perform an exercise breathing count of no less than 7 seconds, and no longer than 10 seconds.

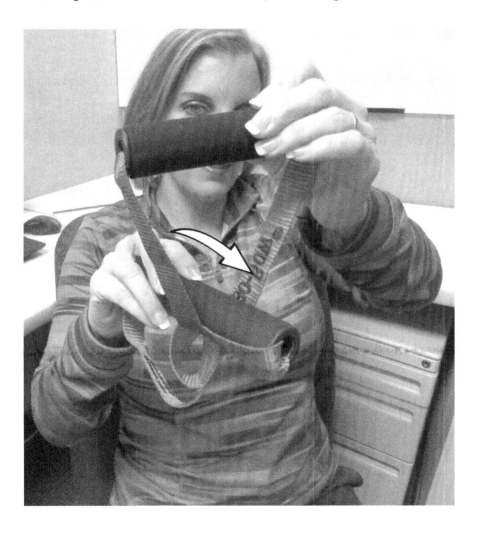

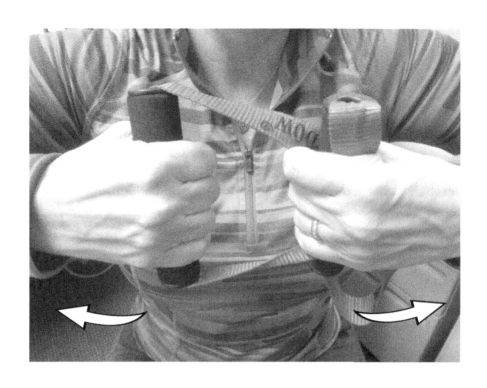

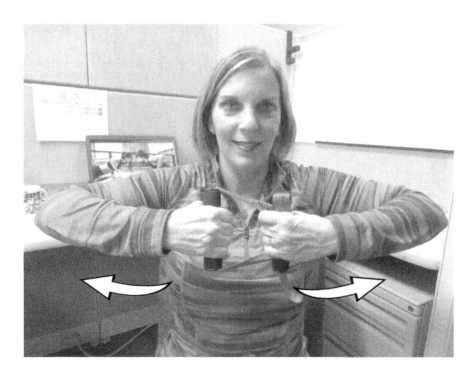

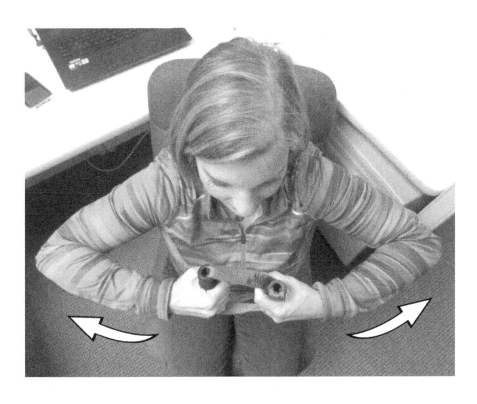

Iso-Bow® Back Power Pull Wide

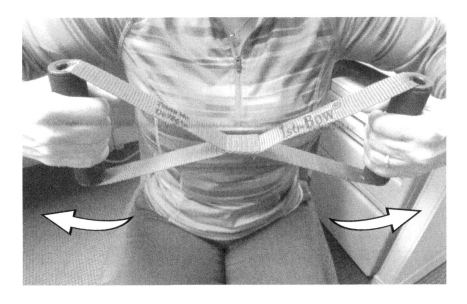

To perform the Iso-Bow® Back Power Pull Wide, hold the Iso-Bow® in front of you, with your arms bent, and approximately parallel to the floor. Attempt to pull the Iso-Bow® apart to engage the upper back muscles. Breathe naturally and deeply in and out for about 10 full breaths, which will take about 1 second per breath. Aim to perform an exercise breathing count of no less than 7 seconds, and no longer than 10 seconds.

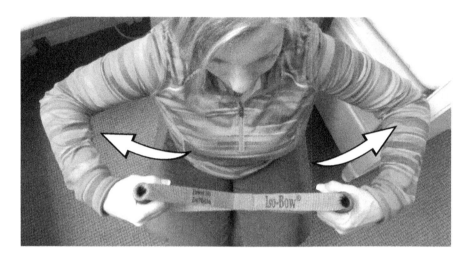

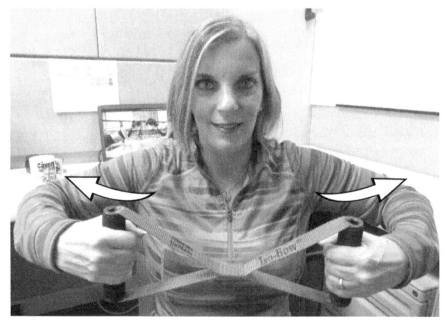

Alternative Exercise Without an Iso-Bow®

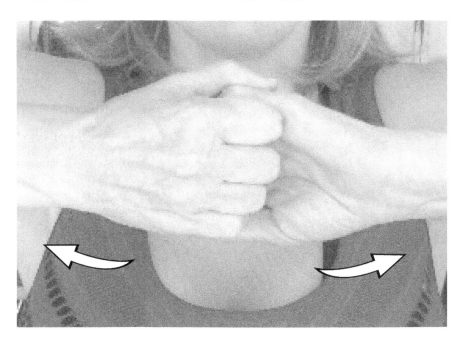

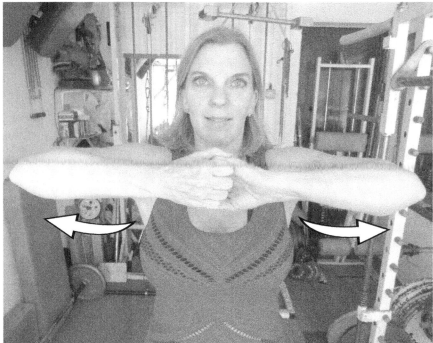

Iso-Bow® Seated Knee Row

Sit on a chair or any other solid object. Bending forwards only from the hips and keeping your back straight.

Lift one knee, and comfortably wrap the Iso-Bow® around it in front of it. Pull back with the handles as you engage your upper back muscles, keeping your elbows close to your body as you do so.

Breathe naturally and deeply in and out for about 10 full breaths, which will take about 1 second per breath.

Aim to perform an exercise breathing count of no less than 7 seconds, and no longer than 10 seconds.

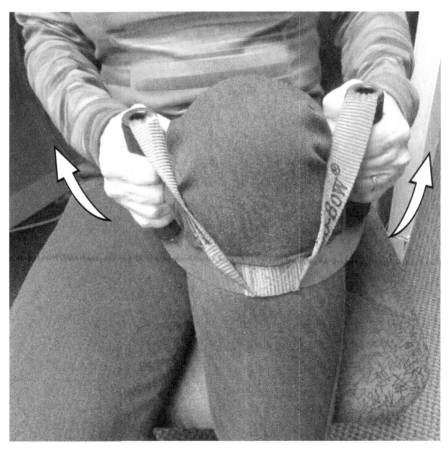

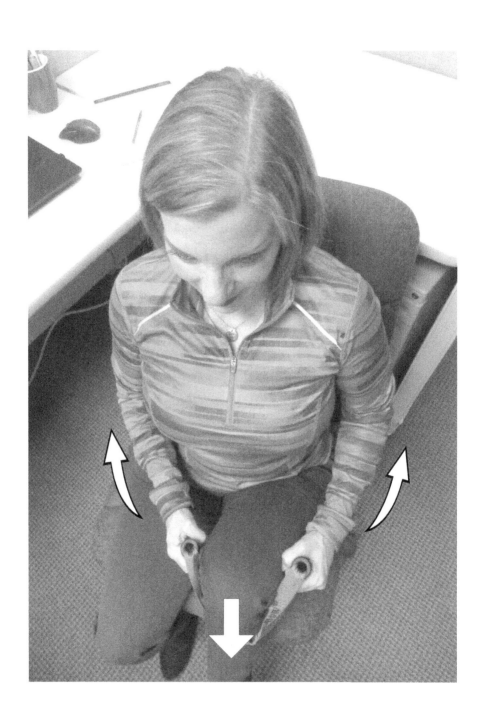

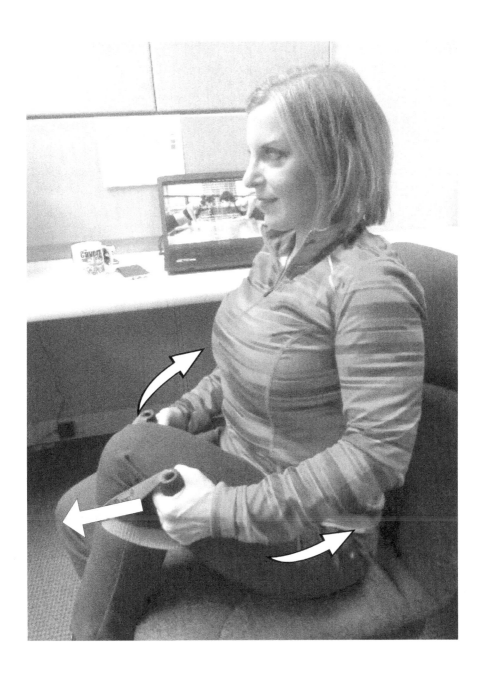

Alternative Exercise Without an Iso-Bow®

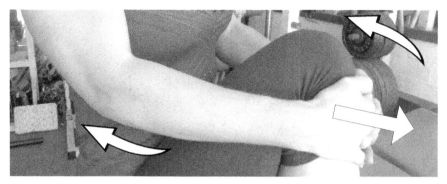

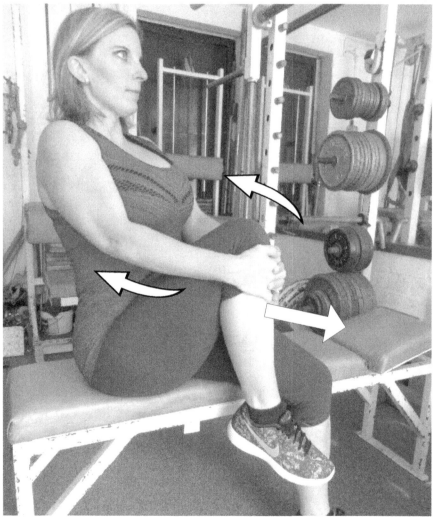

Iso-Bow® Archer Row – Right and Left Side

With one arm in front of you roughly parallel to the floor, push one end of the Iso-Bow® forward. At the same time, pull the other handle backwards to engage the upper back muscles on that side of the body. Breathe naturally and deeply in and out for about 10 full breaths, which will take about 1 second per breath. Aim to perform an exercise breathing count of no less than 7 seconds, and no longer than 10 seconds. Reverse the handgrip positions to exercise the upper back muscles on the other side of your torso.

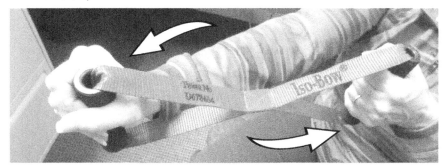

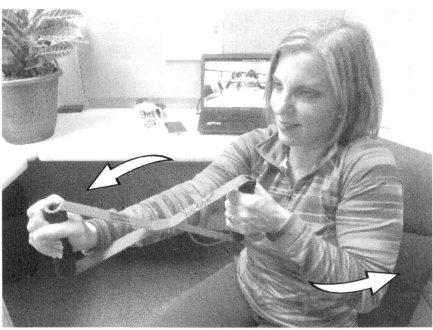

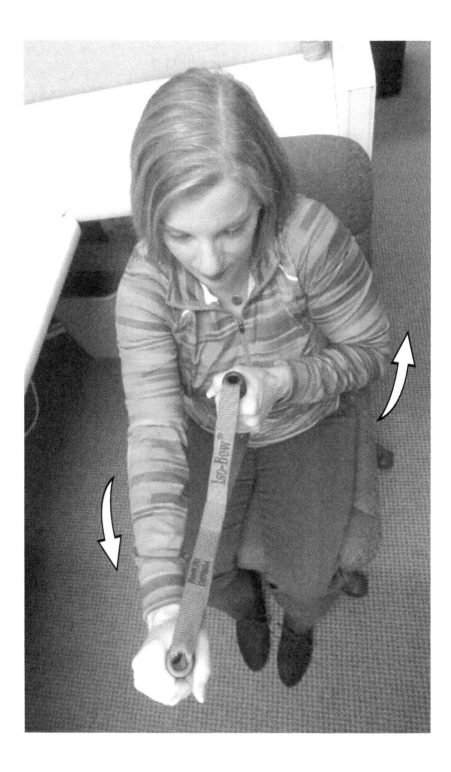

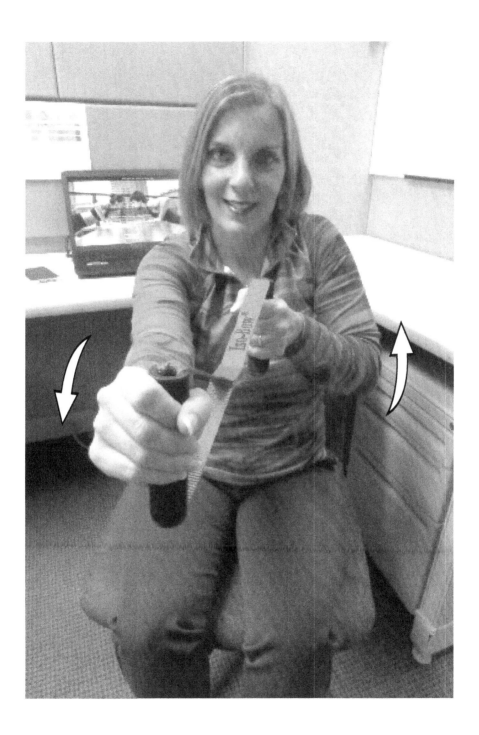

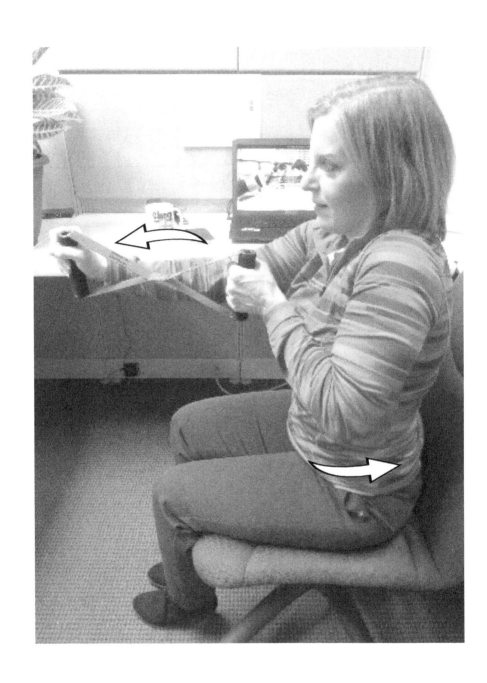

Dual Iso-Bow® Seated Foot Stirrup Row

Sit on a chair or any other solid object, with your feet on the floor in front of you and bend your knees and hips while keeping your back straight. Place one of the looped ends of each Iso-Bow® around each foot, hold the handles firmly, and pull your elbows and arms back to engage your upper back muscles, and be sure to keep your elbows close to your body as you do so. Breathe naturally and deeply in and out for about 10 full breaths, which will take about 1 second per breath. Aim to perform an exercise breathing count of no less than 7 seconds, and no longer than 10 seconds.

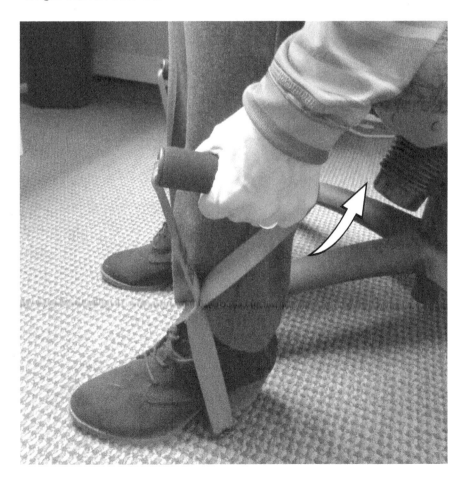

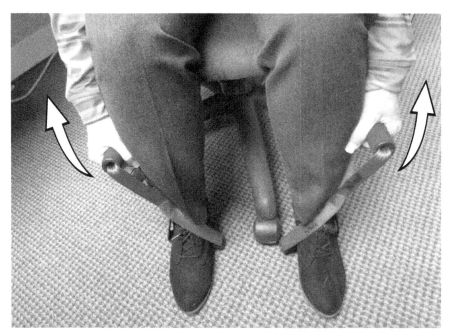

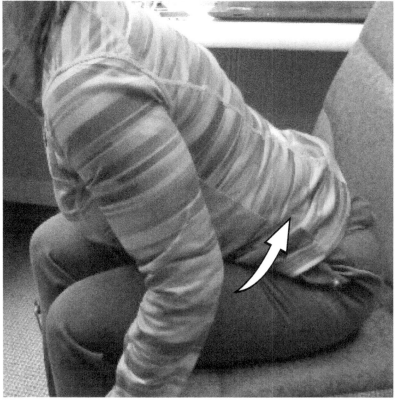

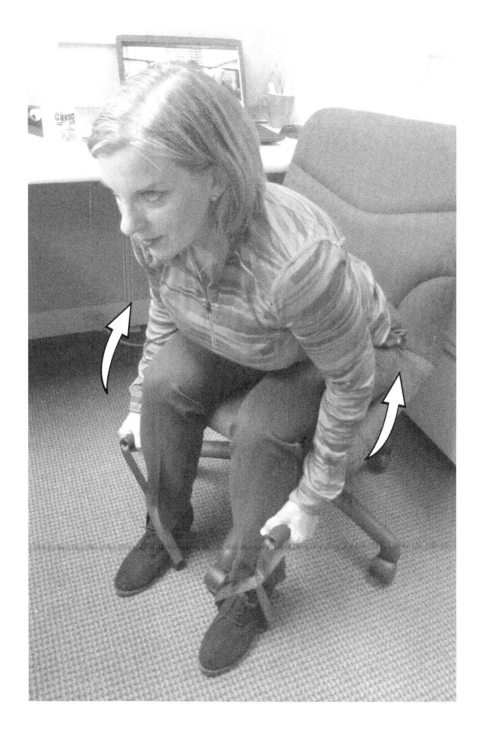

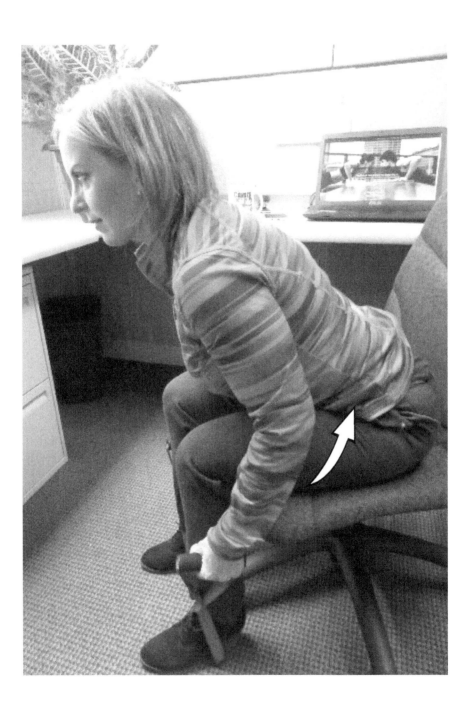

Lower Back: *Dual Iso-Bow® Bent-Leg Deadlift*

Place the loop handle of each Iso-Bow® around each foot as shown. Hold both handles firmly, while maintaining a perfect bent-knee, semi-squat position.

With your back straight, attempt to slowly stand up straight. As you do so, engage the muscles of the glutes, hamstrings, lower back, thighs, and other core muscles. At the same time, the Iso-Bows®, secured by your feet, prevent any further movement from taking place.

Breathe naturally and deeply in and out for about 10 full breaths, which will take about 1 second per breath.

Aim to perform an exercise breathing count of no less than 7 seconds, and no longer than 10 seconds.

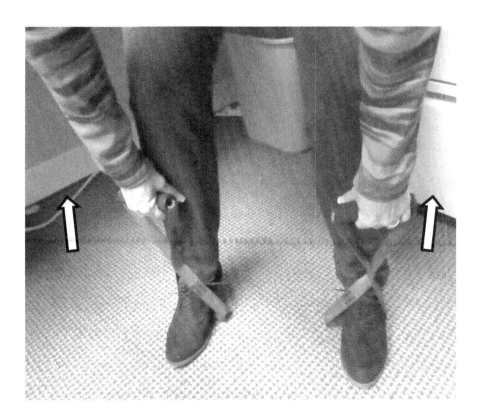

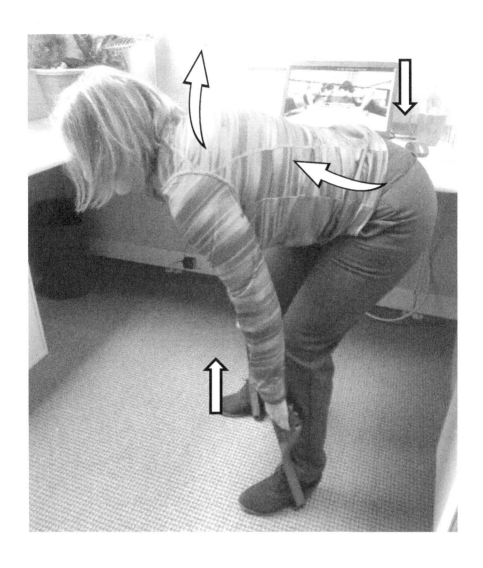

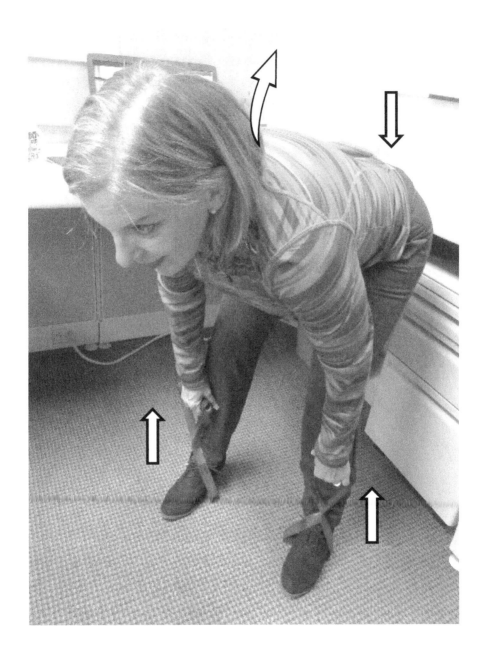

Variation with/from an office chair

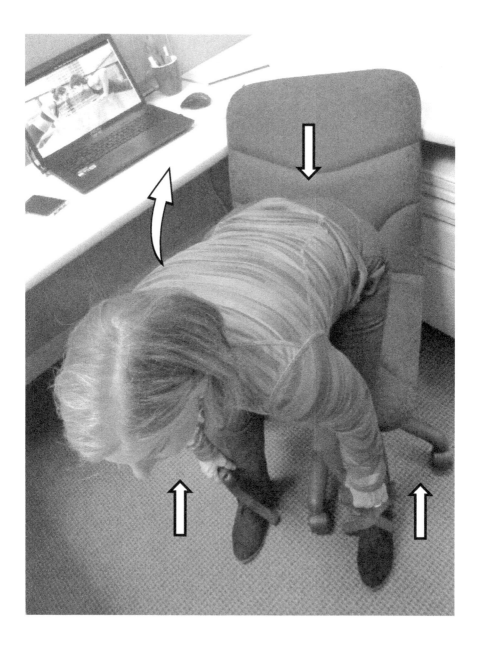

Iso-Bow® Seated Knee Lower Back Press

NOTE: This exercise is performed in the same position as the 'Seated Knee Row' for the upper back. However, some fundamental differences make it a very effective lower-back exercise. Sit on a chair or any other solid object. Bending forwards only from the hips and keeping your back straight. Lift one knee, and comfortably wrap the Iso-Bow® around it in front of it. Instead of pulling back on the handles with the arms so the elbows are close to the body as they perform an upper back exercise, to exercise the lower back muscles, keep the arms locked in a fixed position, or even straight – depending upon how tall you are. Focus on keeping the back straight and pivoting only from the hips as you engage the lower back muscles to try and pull your knee back. To counterbalance this, your knee presses forward so that an isometric exercise is performed for the lower back muscles. Ideally, perform the same exercise using both knees. Breathe naturally and deeply in and out for about 10 full breaths, which will take about 1 second per breath. Aim to perform an exercise breathing count of no less than 7 seconds, and no longer than 10 seconds.

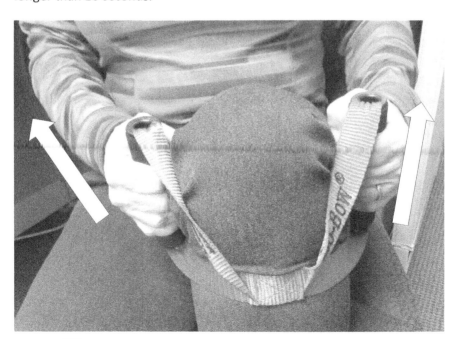

The upright line demonstrates the upright torso position with the back straight. The line and arrow to the right demonstrate the direction in which force is applied by engaging the muscles of the lower back.

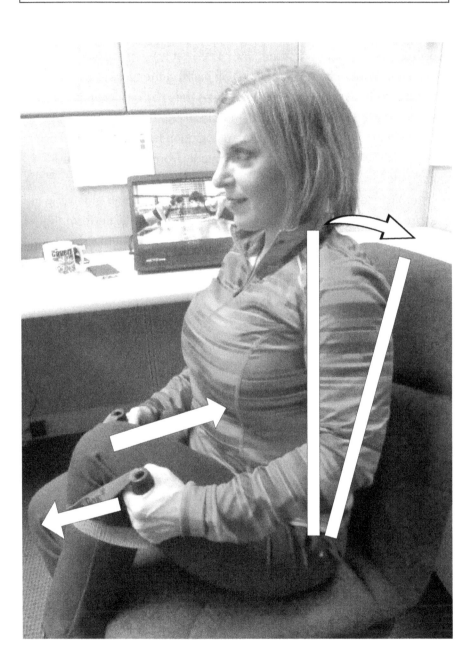

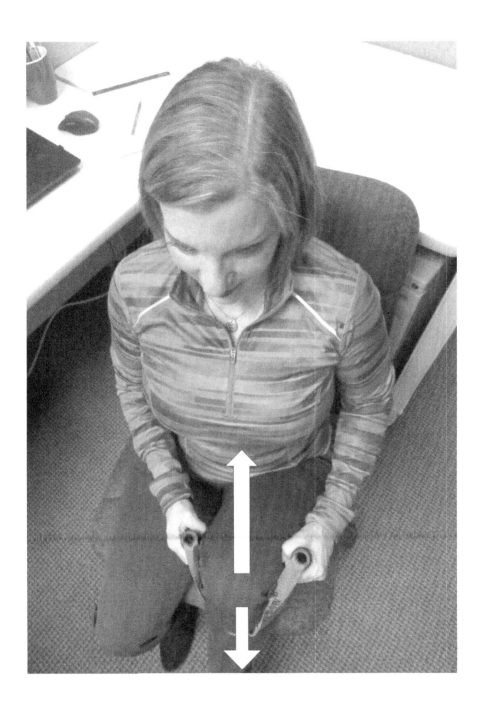

Alternative Exercise Without an Iso-Bow®

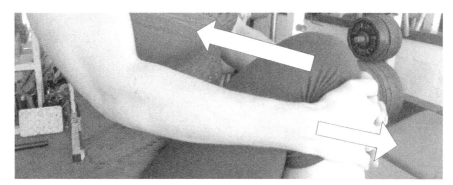

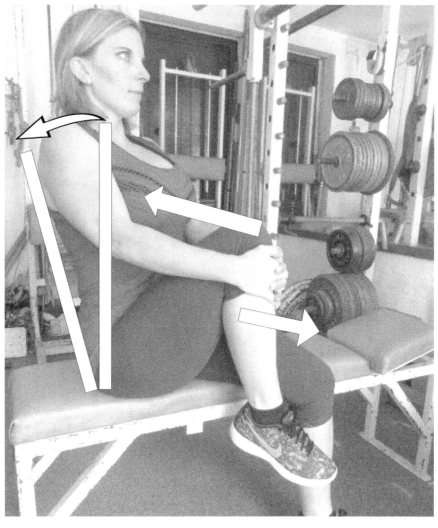

Chest: Iso-Bow® Cradle Cross Press

Cradle the Iso-Bow® to make a shorter handgrip. Cross it in front of you at chest level, with your arms roughly parallel to the floor, and push in opposing directions sideways to engage your chest muscles.

Breathe naturally and deeply in and out for about 10 full breaths, which will take about 1 second per breath. Aim to perform an exercise breathing count of no less than 7 seconds, and no longer than 10 seconds.

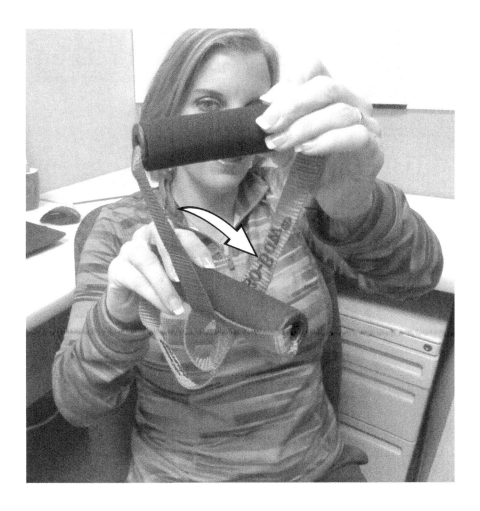

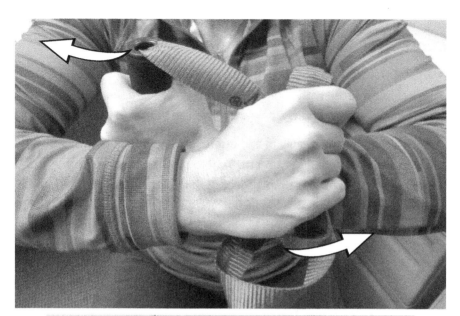

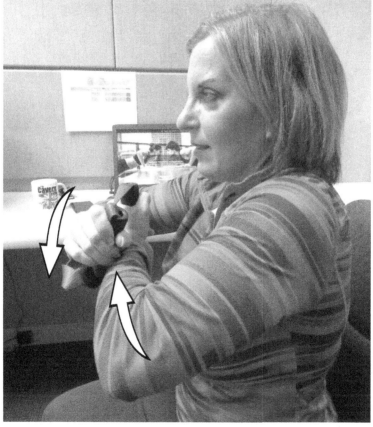

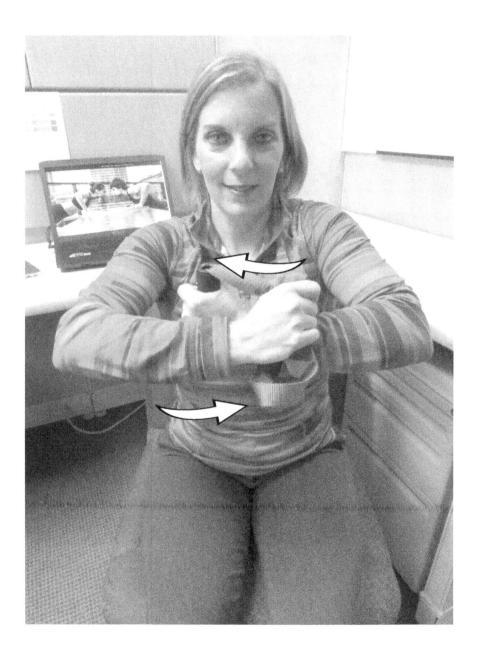

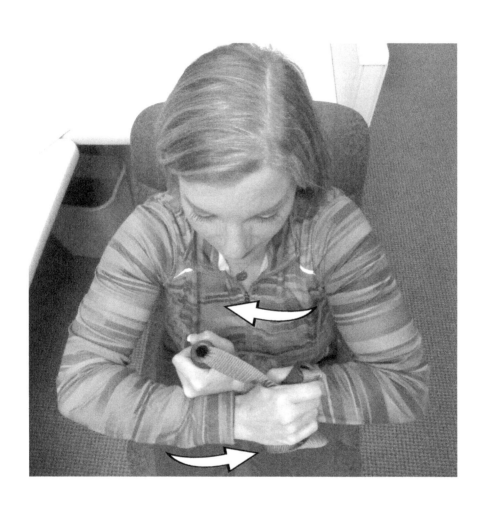

Iso-Bow® Chest Cross Press Wide

Cross the Iso-Bow® in front of you at chest level, with your arms roughly parallel to the floor. Push in opposing directions sideways, to engage your chest muscles.

Breathe naturally and deeply in and out for about 10 full breaths, which will take about 1 second per breath.

Aim to perform an exercise breathing count of no less than 7 seconds, and no longer than 10 seconds.

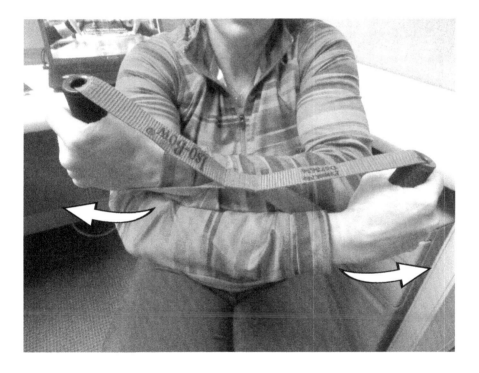

169

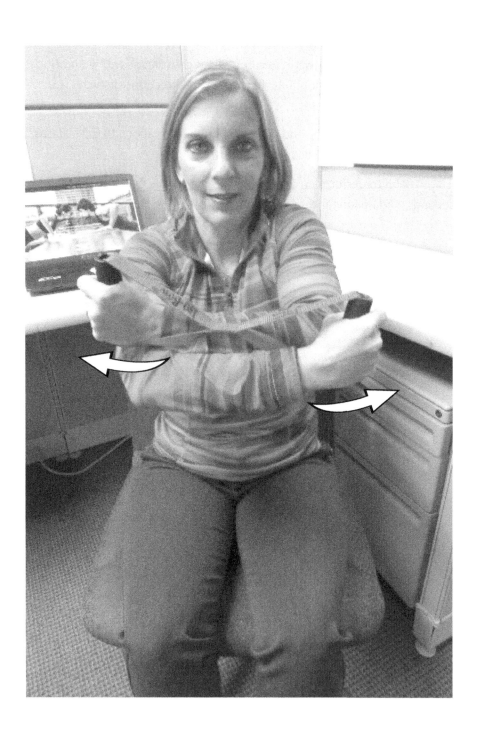

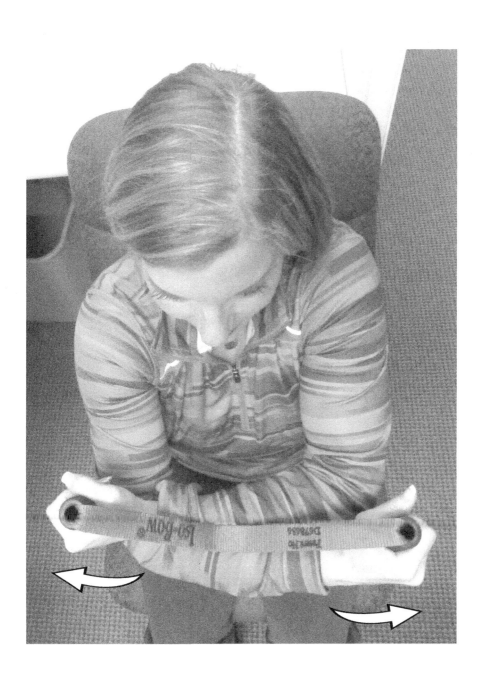

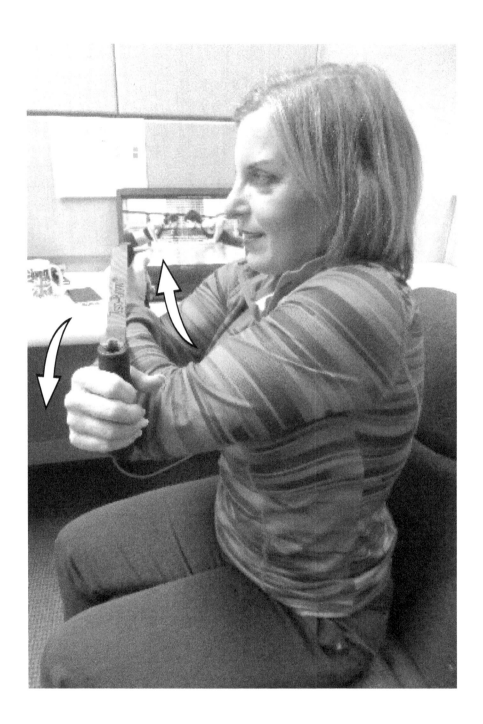

Iso-Bow® Chest Press Inner and Outer Push

With one arm in front of you roughly parallel to the floor, push one end of the Iso-Bow® forward. As you do so, keep your elbow slightly bent, and focus your push slightly inwards, across to the centre point of the chest. At the same time, push the other handle inwards, and across your chest. This exercise should engage the inner and outer chest muscles at the same time. Always keep the elbows of both arms slightly during the exercise. Breathe naturally and deeply in and out for about 10 full breaths, which will take about 1 second per breath. Aim to perform an exercise breathing count of no less than 7 seconds, and no longer than 10 seconds. Reverse the handgrip positions to exercise the inner and outer portions of the chest on the other side of your torso.

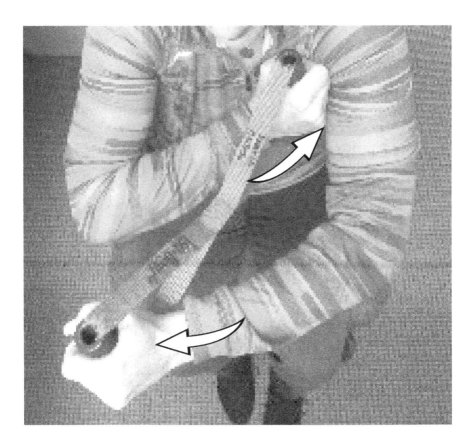

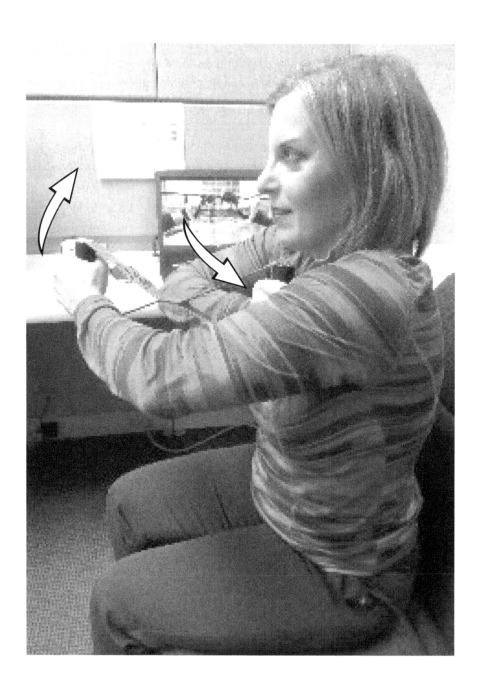

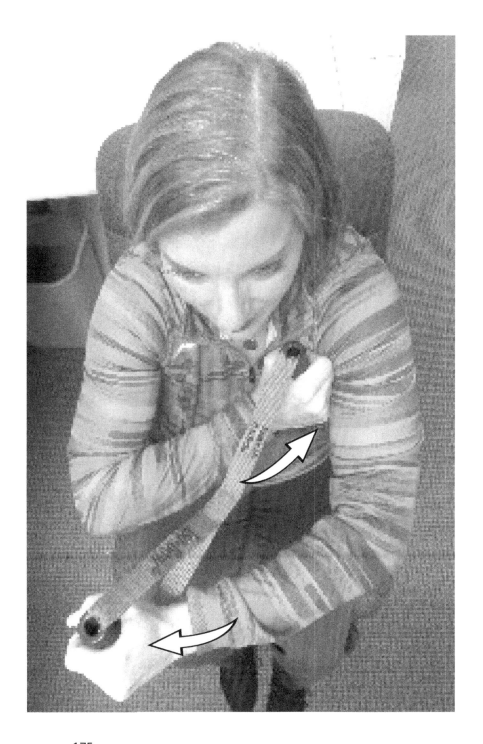

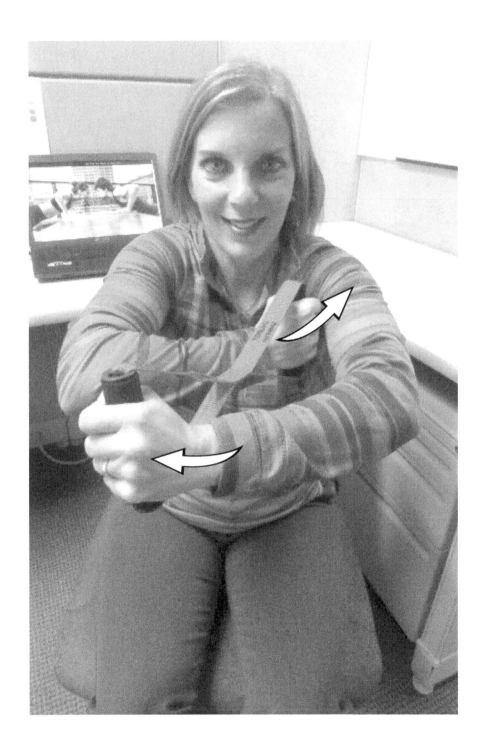

Alternative Chest Exercise Without an Iso-Bow®

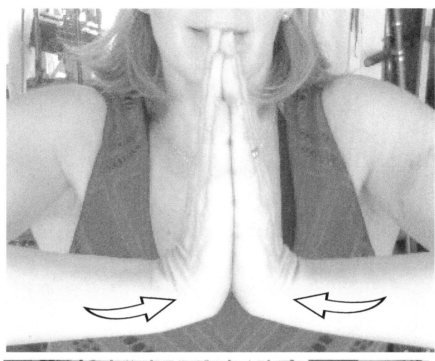

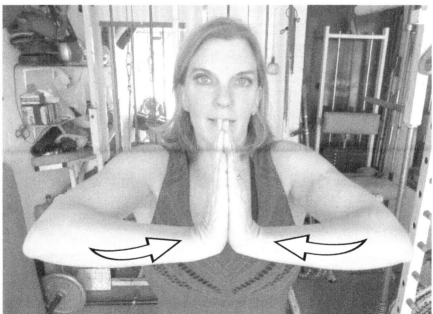

Shoulders:
Iso-Bow® Overhead Press – Left and Right Arm

Hold one end of the Iso-Bow® in your upper hand, ensuring that your arm always stays at an angle of approximately 90 degrees. Push upwards, as if to perform a shoulder press, and resist the movement by pulling back and downwards with the opposing hand and arm. Breathe naturally and deeply in and out for about 10 full breaths, which will take about 1 second per breath. Aim to perform an exercise breathing count of no less than 7 seconds, and no longer than 10 seconds. Then repeat the exercise on the other side for the other shoulder.

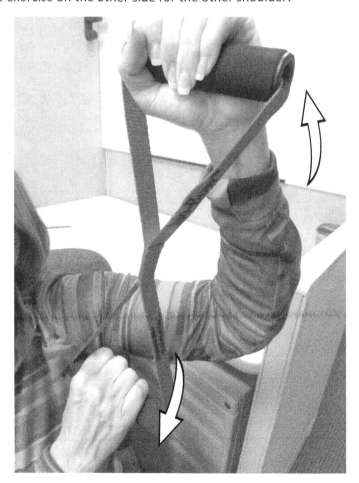

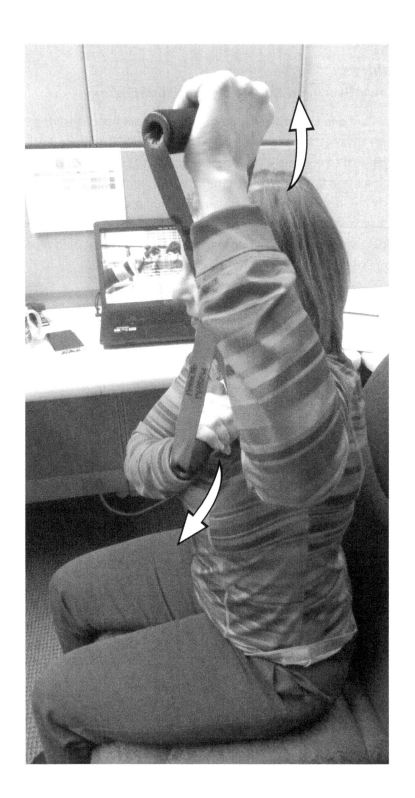

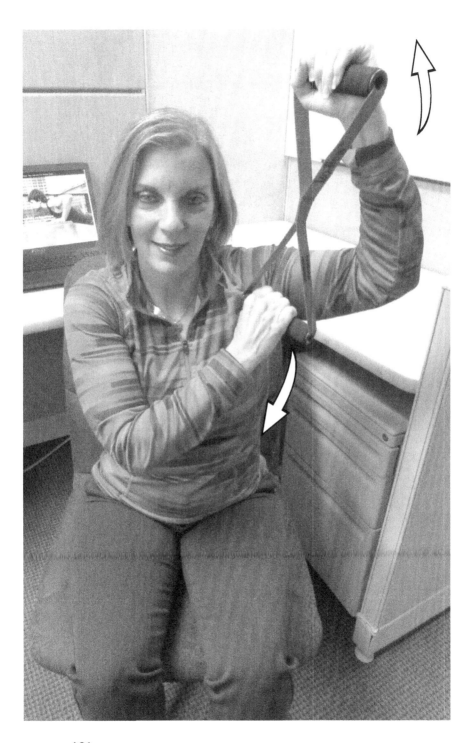

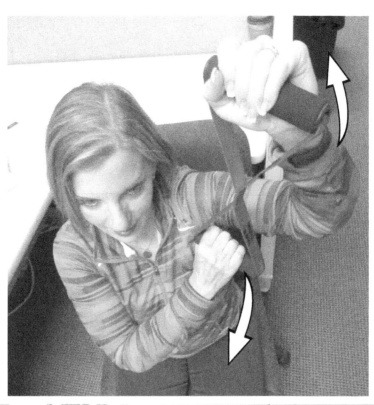

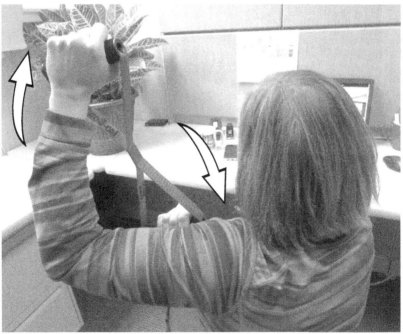

Iso-Bow® Front Raise - Left and Right Arm

Standing upright, hold the Iso-Bow® in front of you as shown, with the palms of both hands facing down.

Keeping both elbows slightly bent, use the front shoulder muscles of the upper arm to resist the downward pull of the lower hand and arm.

Breathe naturally and deeply in and out for about 10 full breaths, which will take about 1 second per breath.

Aim to perform an exercise breathing count of no less than 7 seconds, and no longer than 10 seconds. Repeat the exercise on the other side by reversing the hand and arm positions.

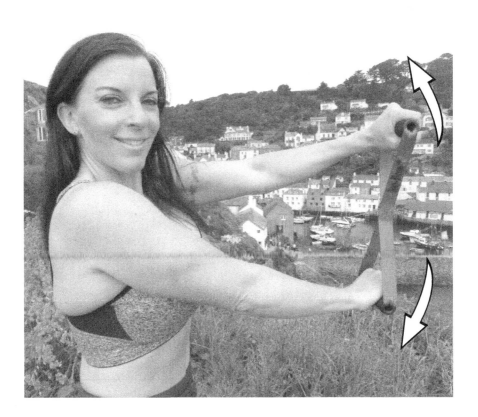

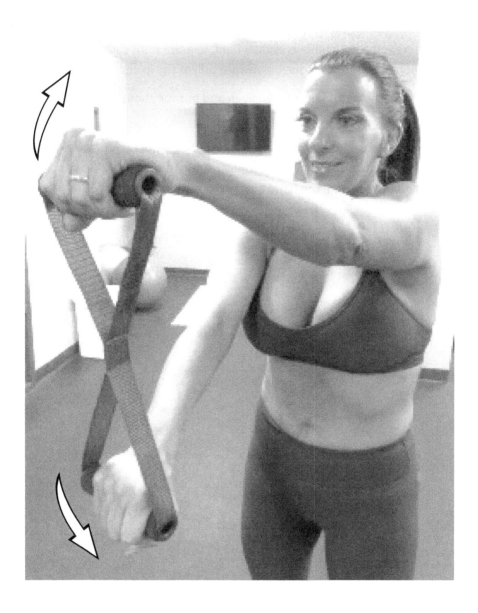

Opposite Arms and Shoulders

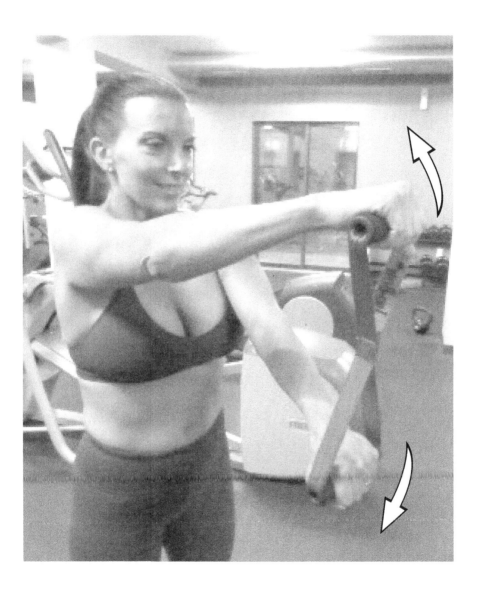

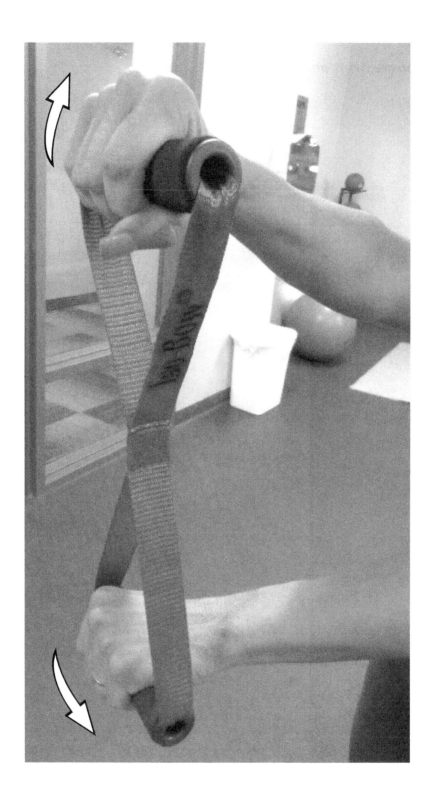

Iso-Bow® Mid Lateral Pull-Apart (Lateral Raise)

Hold the Iso-Bow® in both hands, at lap level in front of you, and with your elbows very slightly bent.

In this position, attempt to pull it apart by raising both arms sideways, and engaging the side shoulder muscles as you do so.

Breathe naturally and deeply in and out for about 10 full breaths, which will take about 1 second per breath.

Aim to perform an exercise breathing count of no less than 7 seconds, and no longer than 10 seconds.

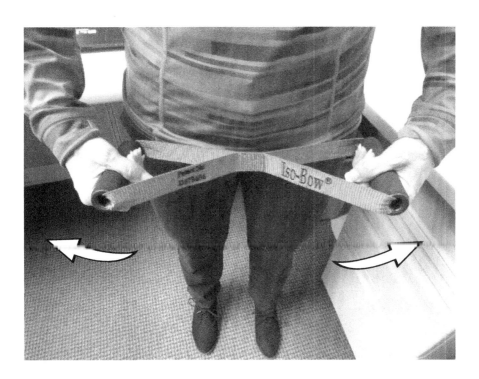

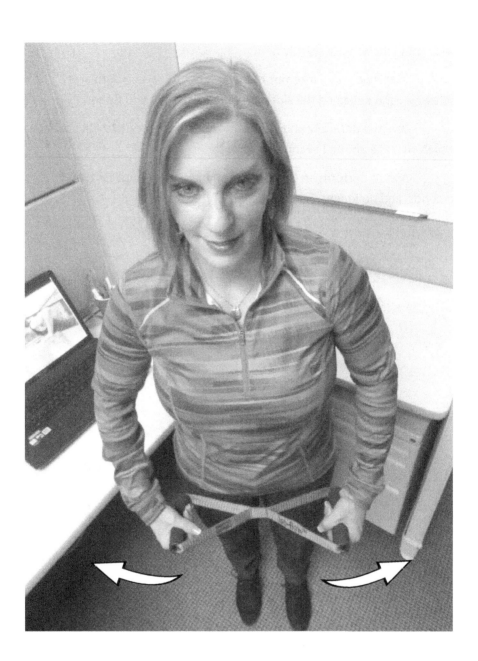

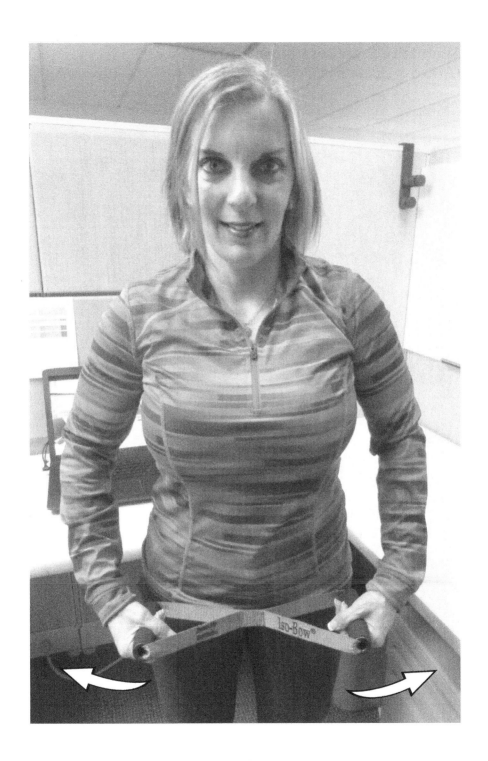

Alternative Exercises Without an Iso-Bow®
(To Exercise Both Shoulders, Change Leading Hand to Other Side)

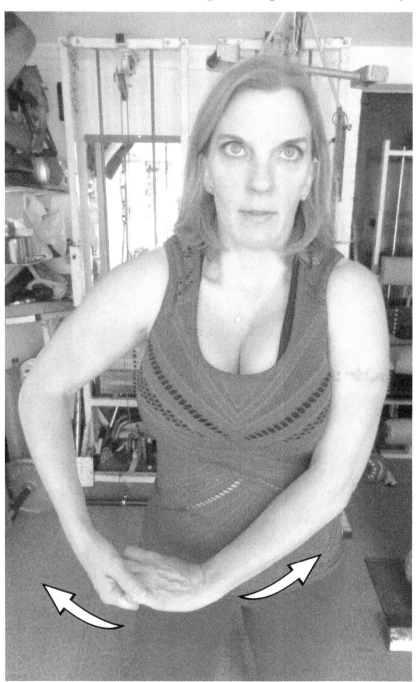

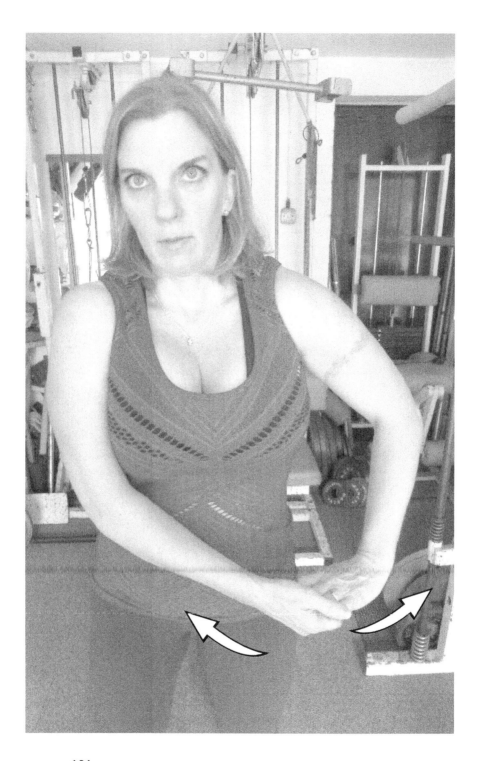

Legs: Upper Thighs
Iso-Bow® Leg Extension – Left and Right Leg

Sit on a chair or any other solid object, raise one knee and place the Iso-Bow® comfortably around the lower part of your leg, close to your foot. Hold both handles firmly, keep your back straight, bend only from the hips, and lean back slightly as you try to extend your foot forward while keeping your toes pointing upwards. Breathe naturally and deeply in and out for about 10 full breaths, which will take about 1 second per breath. Aim to perform an exercise breathing count of no less than 7 seconds, and no longer than 10 seconds. Switch legs and repeat the exercise with the other leg. As an alternative to using your lower shin to resist the Iso-Bow®, you can equally easily loop one foot, through one handle of each Iso-Bow® as shown. Keeping your toes pulled upwards, engage the thigh muscles by applying pressure to extend the foot forwards, and slightly upwards.

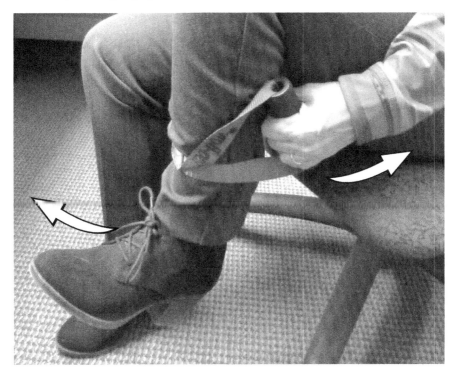

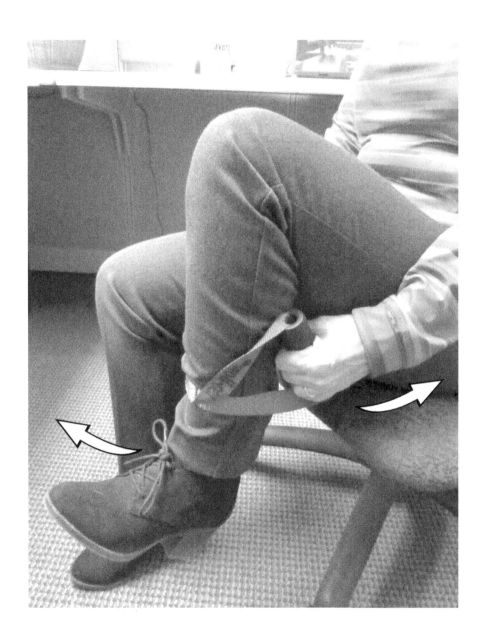

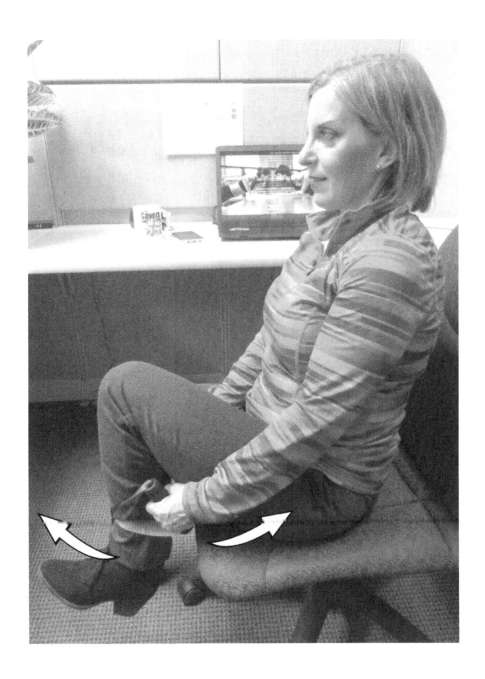

Alternative Exercise With Foot Loop Iso-Bow®

As an alternative to using your lower shin to resist the Iso-Bow®, you can equally easily loop one foot, through one handle of each Iso-Bow® as shown. Keeping your toes pulled upwards, engage the thigh muscles by applying pressure to extend the foot forwards, and slightly upwards.

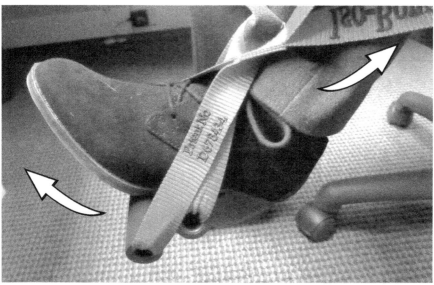

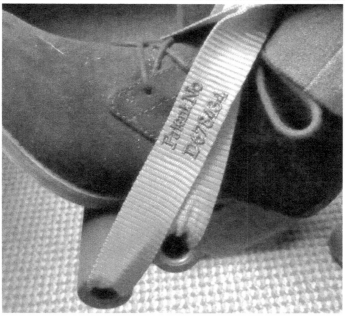

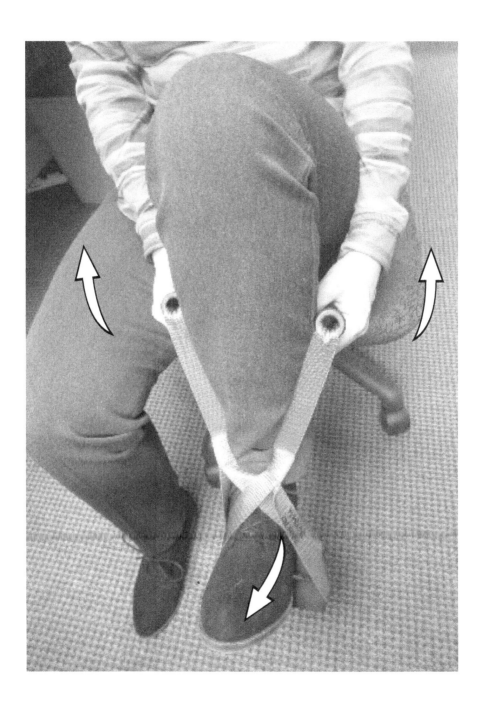

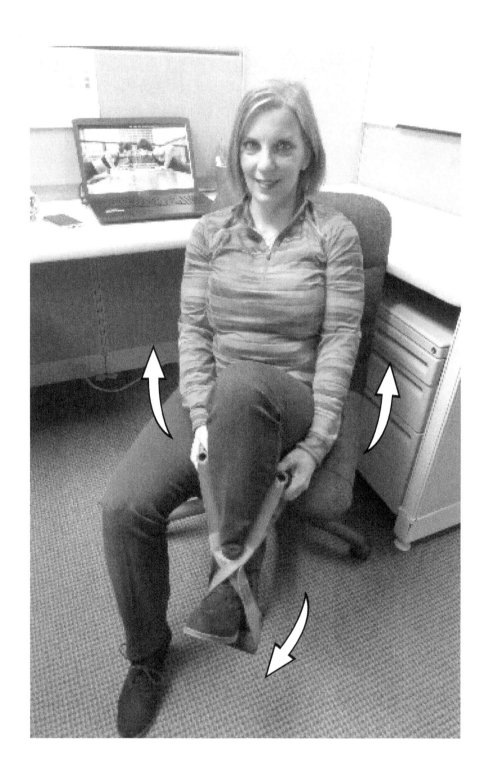

Alternative Exercise Without an Iso-Bow®

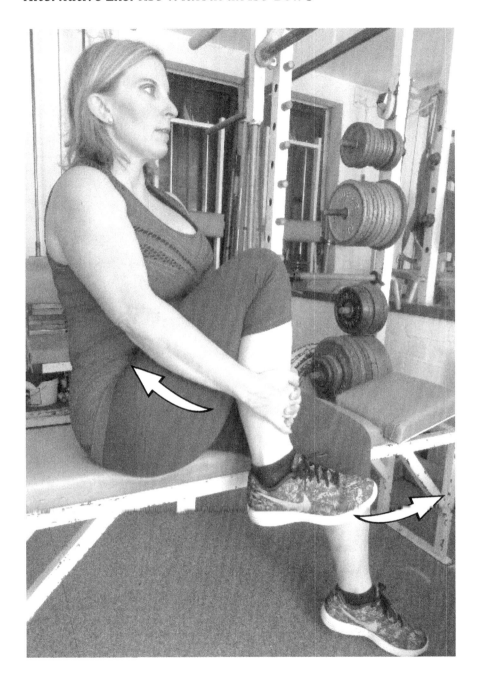

Iso-Bow® Hamstring Seated Curl and Extension – Both Legs

Sit on a chair or any other solid object and push the Iso-Bow® comfortably down over one leg to help prevent it from rising during the exercise.

Place one foot directly in front of the other, so the heel of the leading foot is touching the toes of your rear foot and turn up the toes to create a firmer connection.

Draw back the leading foot by engaging the hamstring muscles of the rear upper thigh, while the rear foot stops it from moving.   Breathe naturally and deeply in and out for about 10 full breaths, which will take about 1 second per breath.

Aim to perform an exercise breathing count of no less than 7 seconds, and no longer than 10 seconds. Repeat the exercise for the other leg, by swapping the leg and foot positions.

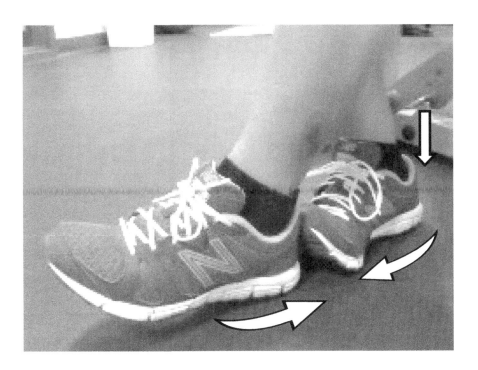

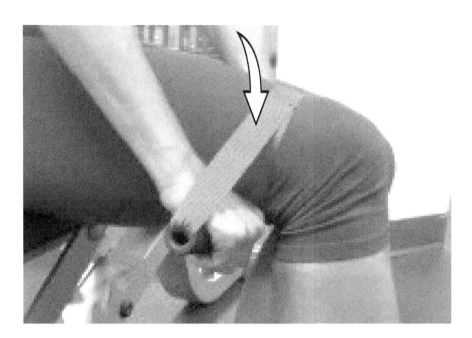

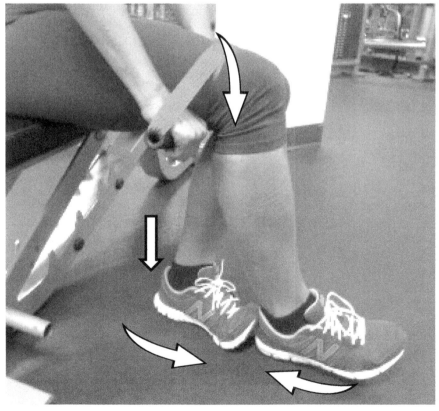

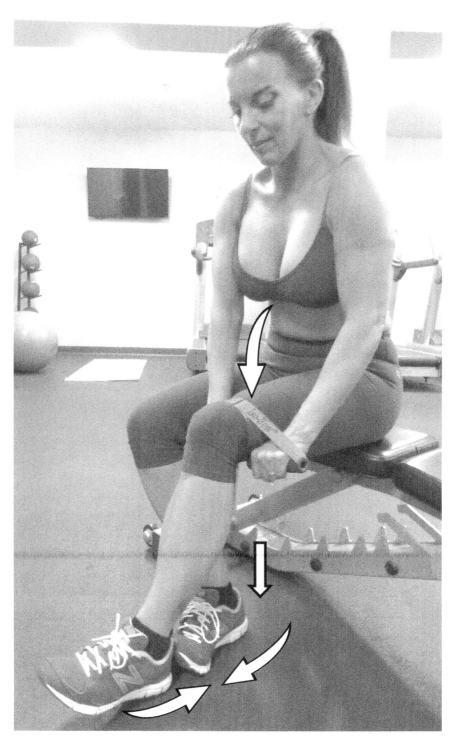

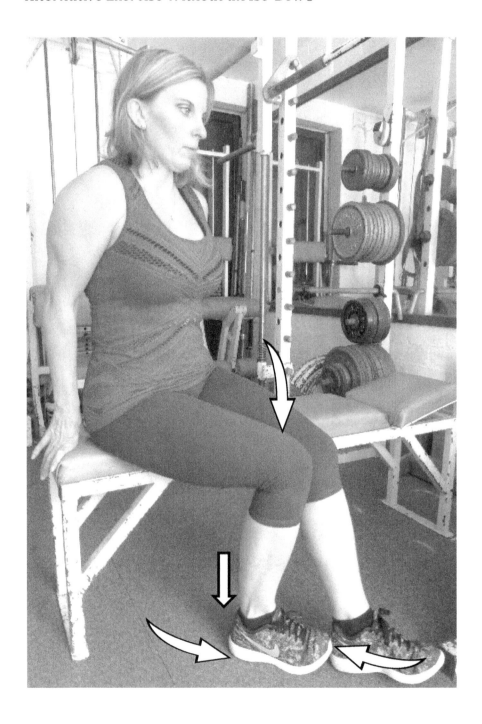

Alternative Exercise
Wall or Door Standing Hamstring Curl

To perform the wall or door hamstring curl, stand with your feet slightly away from a wall or other solid object. In this position, raise one leg slightly to the rear so that the heel meets the wall/object. Always keep your foot and toes pulled up and toward your knee. With your back flat against the wall, attempt to curl your leg by pushing the heel into the wall and upwards to perform the exercise. Do not forget the other leg.

When you perform an isometric exercise never hold your breath. Always breathe deeply and naturally, which will be about 10 full breaths at a rate of about 1 second per breath. Perform each exercise for no less than 7 seconds, and no longer than 10

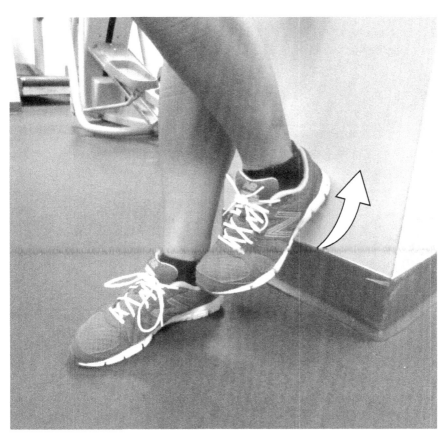

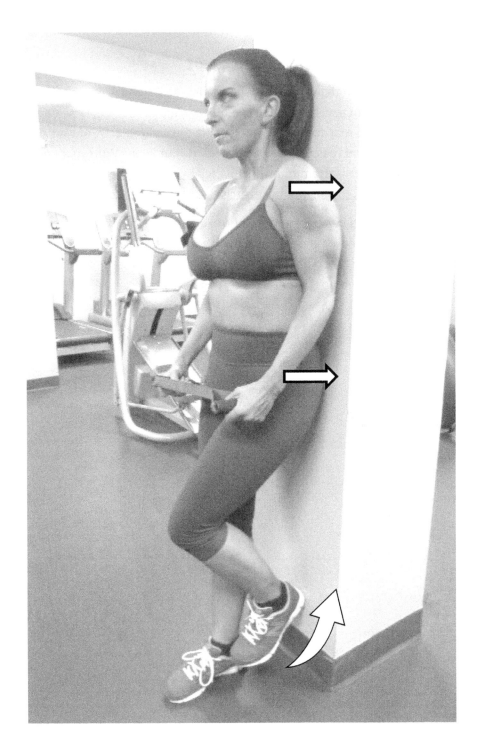

Iso-Bow® Foot Loop Abductor

Place each of the Iso-Bow® handles around your feet as shown and lean back on a chair.

Lift your legs slightly off the floor, and pull your feet apart, sideways to engage the outer thigh, hip, and glute muscles.

Breathe naturally and deeply in and out for about 10 full breaths, which will take about 1 second per breath.

Aim to perform an exercise breathing count of no less than 7 seconds, and no longer than 10 seconds.

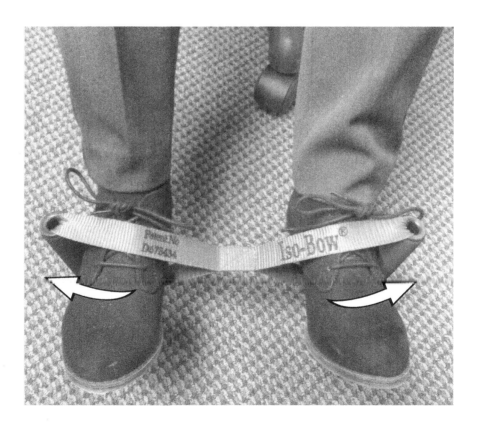

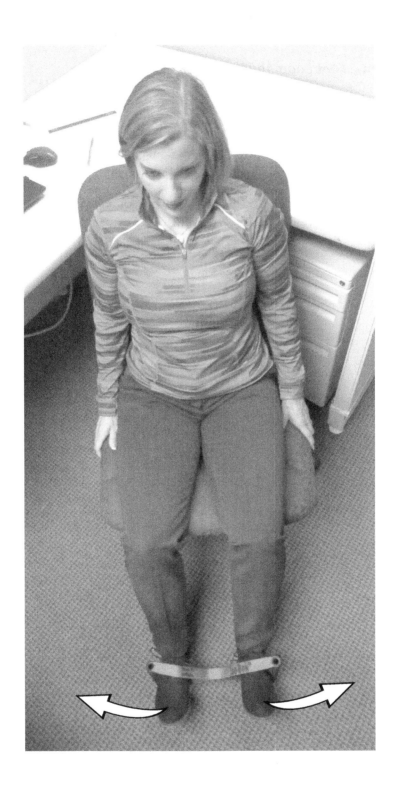

Iso-Bow® Knee Hold Abductor

Sit on a chair or any other solid object and place the Iso-Bow® around the knees as shown.

Hold the handles as you attempt to pull the knees apart to engage the outer thigh muscles and the glutes.

Breathe naturally and deeply in and out for about 10 full breaths, which will take about 1 second per breath.

Aim to perform an exercise breathing count of no less than 7 seconds, and no longer than 10 seconds.

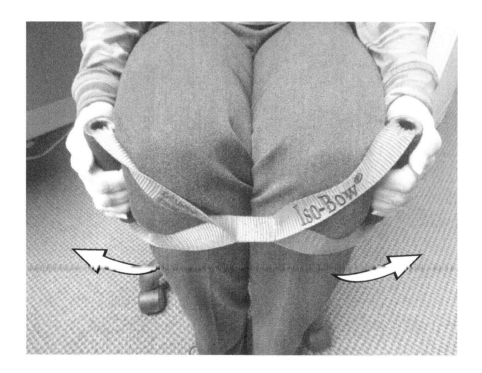

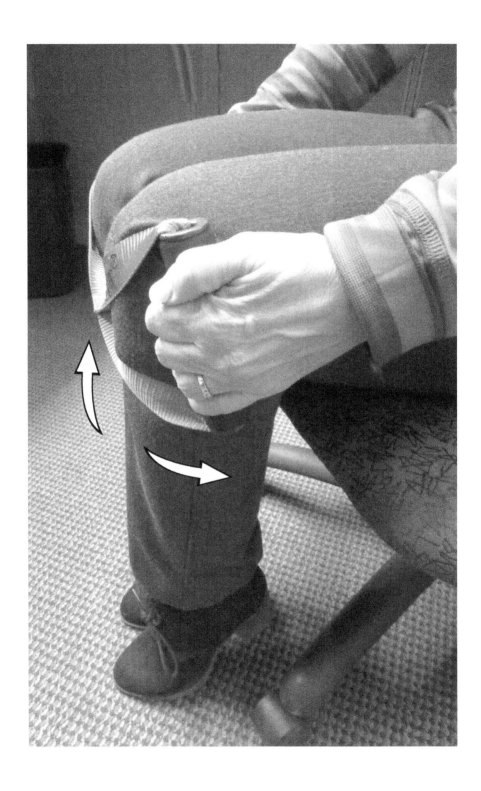

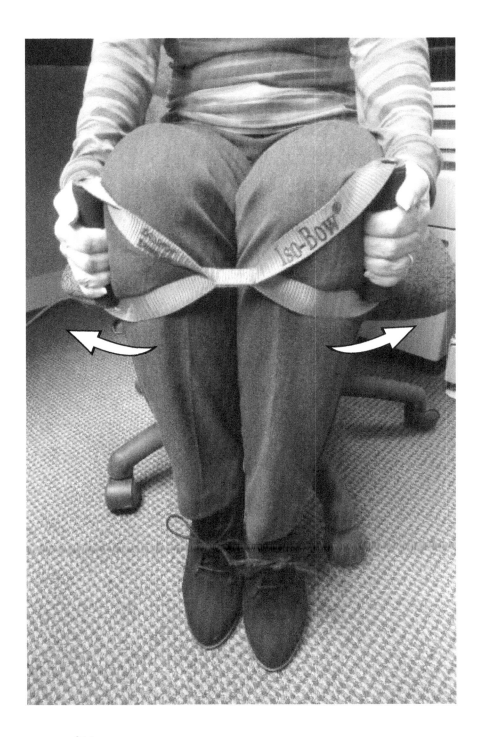

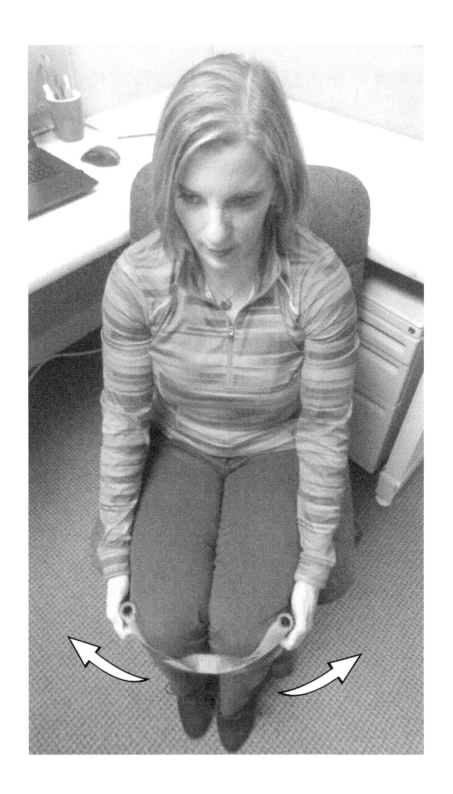

Iso-Bow® Knee-Press Adductor

Sit on a chair or any other solid object. Wrap two Iso-Bows® together to make a four-handle pair, then place them between the knees. Squeeze the knees together to engage the two Iso-Bows® with inner thigh muscles. Breathe naturally and deeply in and out for about 10 full breaths, which will take about 1 second per breath. Aim to perform an exercise breathing count of no less than 7 seconds, and no longer than 10 seconds.

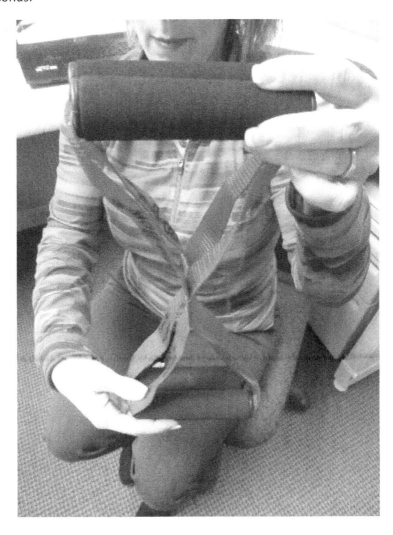

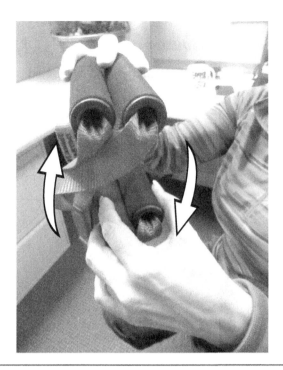

Wrap one end of a single Iso-Bow®, or pair, tightly around the other end to form a secure non-slip bundle grip.

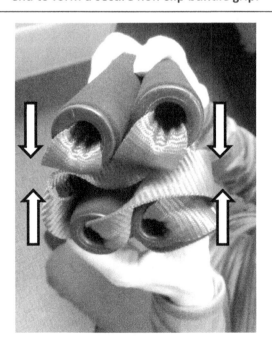

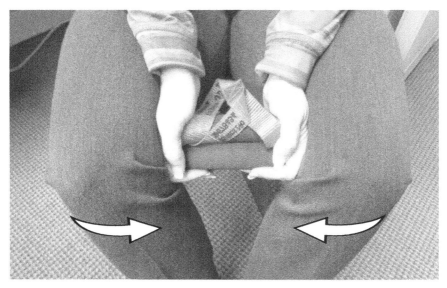

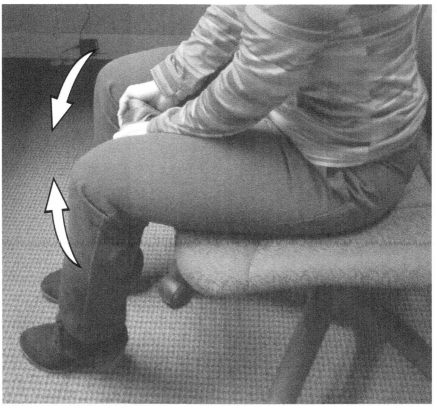

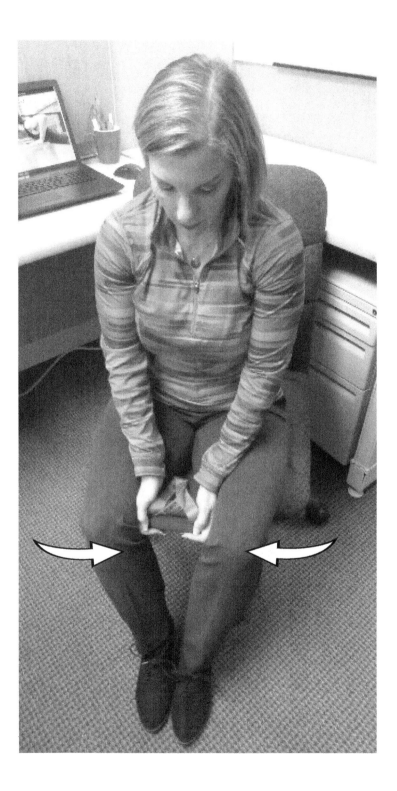

Dual Iso-Bow® Stirrup Squat

Place one looped handle side of each Iso-Bow® around each foot as shown. Bend your torso forward and only at the hips, always keeping your back straight and upright. Grip each Iso-Bow® handle firmly and attempt to stand upright from your chair by engaging your upper thigh and glute muscles. You can always perform this exercise without a chair, by starting in the standing position. Naturally, you will not be able to move but continue your attempt to stand up, while maintaining the perfect mid-squat position as you do so. Breathe naturally and deeply in and out for about 10 full breaths, which will take about 1 second per breath. Aim to perform an exercise breathing count of no less than 7 seconds, and no longer than 10 seconds.

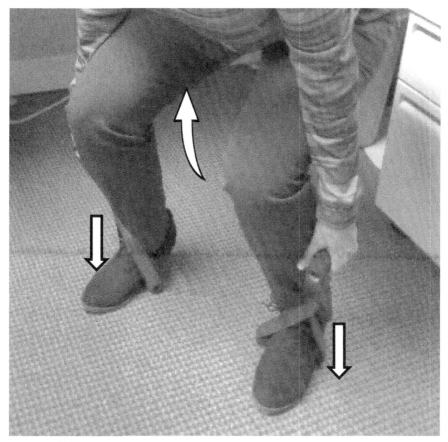

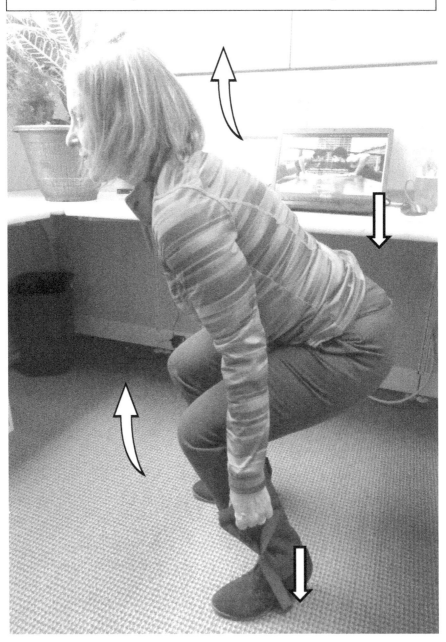

NOTE: To secure each Iso-Bow® with the feet, either step into it so the lower handle is in the shoe recess between the sole and heel or move the lower handle to one side to allow the foot to sit in the stirrup it creates and sit flat on the strap.

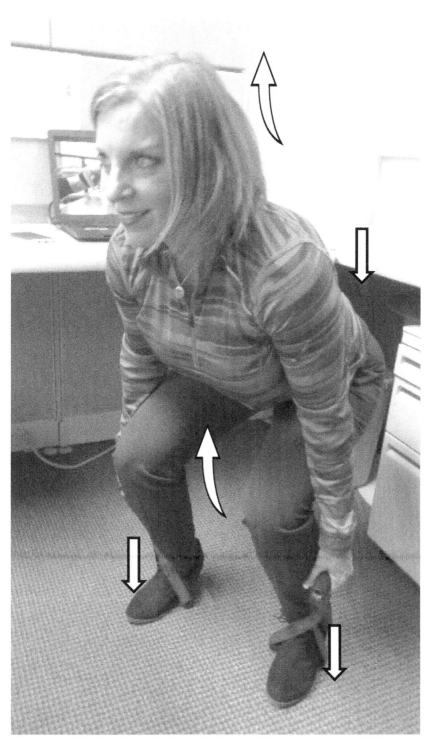

Alternative Sitting up from or Over a Chair – 2 Iso-Bows®

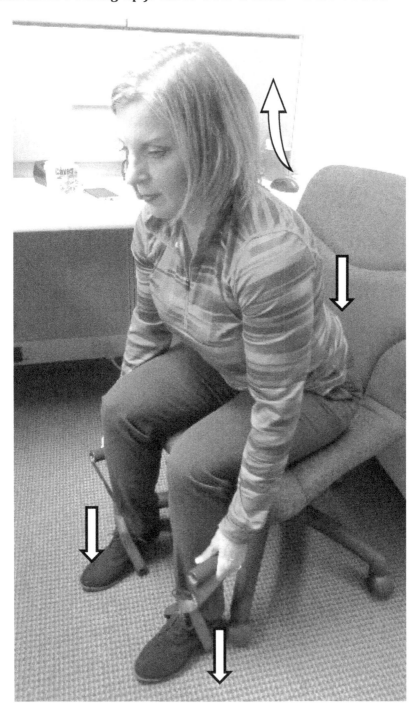

Squat Hover-Hold - Over a Chair

With the feet approximately shoulder-width apart and the back straight, attempt to slowly stand upright from a seated position on a chair. If possible, do so without using your arms to help. When your body is just off the chair, hold that position by using your thighs and buttocks to do so. Breathe naturally and deeply in and out for about 10 full breaths, which will take about 1 second per breath. Aim to perform an exercise breathing count of no less than 7 seconds, and no longer than 10 seconds.

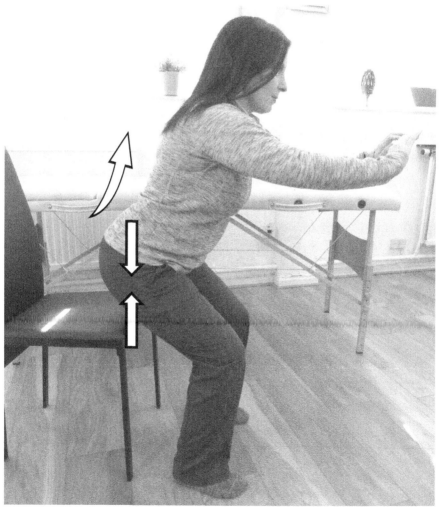

Alternative Exercise
Door or Wall Squat Isometric Press

Use either a wall or a suitable closed and locked door that cannot be opened accidentally. Stand with your back to it, squat down and lean against it until your legs are bent at about 90 degrees. Keep your torso upright and your feet about shoulder-width apart. In this position, push back against the door, and also slightly upwards, as if attempting to lift the door or wall. You can then begin performing an isometric exercise. Always breathe deeply and naturally as you perform the exercise, which will be about 10 full breaths, at a rate of about 1 second per breath. Perform the exercise for no less than 7 seconds, and no longer than 10.

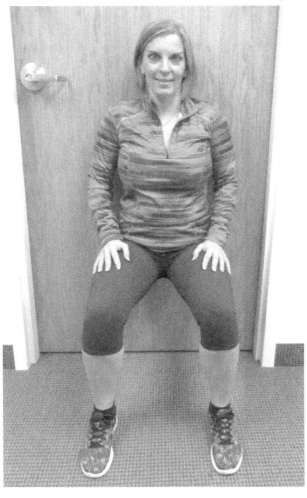

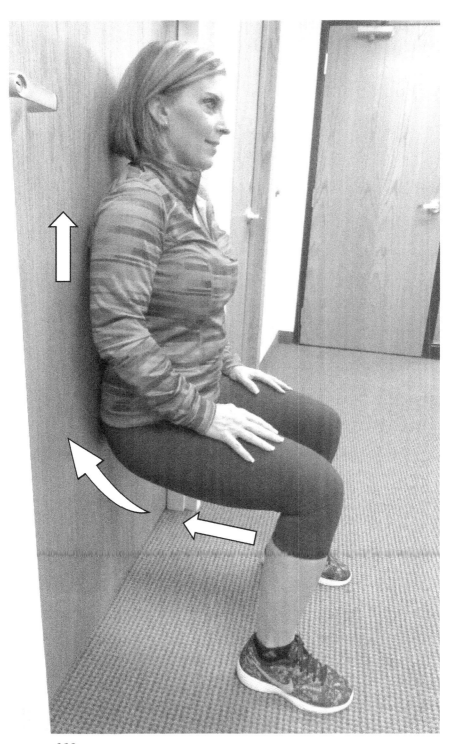

223

Legs: Calf's

Calf Single Leg Wall Push – Left and Right Leg

Place your hands against a wall, a door and/or frame, or any other solid object which is immovable by human muscle power alone.

With one leg back in a firm position, with the ball of your foot firmly on the floor, raise the heel slightly as you engage your calf muscles, pushing against the immovable object.

Breathe naturally and deeply in and out for about 10 full breaths, which will take about 1 second per breath.

Aim to perform an exercise breathing count of no less than 7 seconds, and no longer than 10 seconds. Switch legs and repeat the exercise with the other leg.

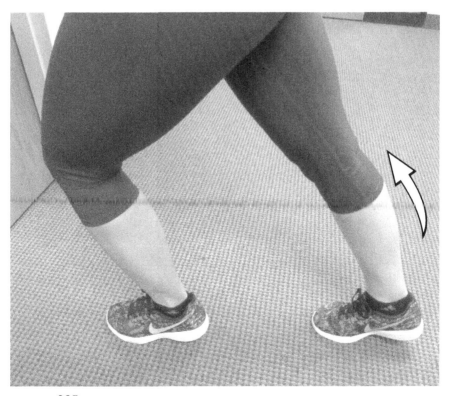

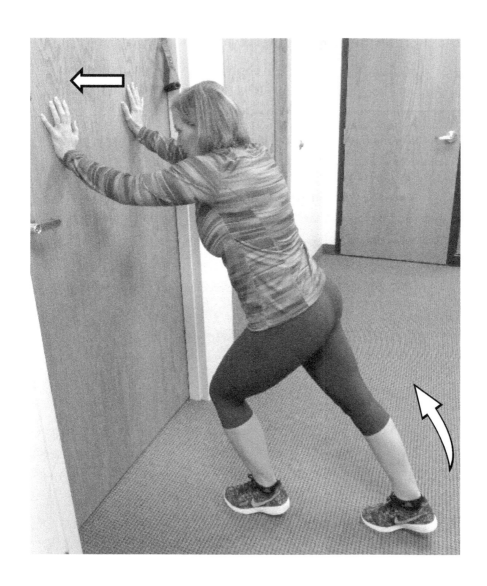

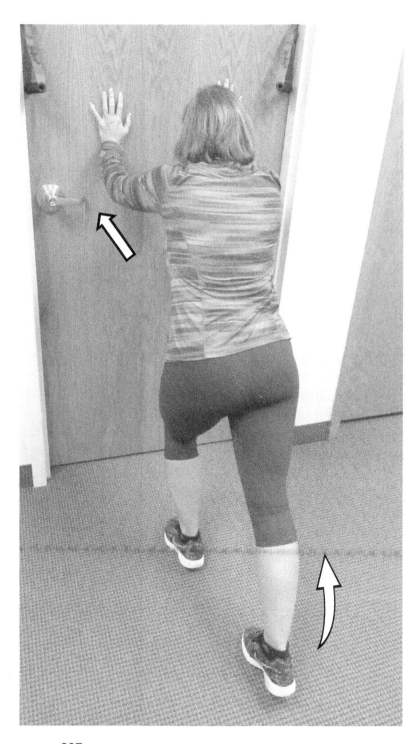

Chapter 9: Conclusion

The advanced isometric exercises the core of the Workout at Work™ concept have been thoroughly researched and proven in independent university studies all around the world. The results of these studies conclusively proved that even one properly performed 7-second isometric exercise can stimulate significant muscle growth, increase strength, and improve muscle tone.

The isometric exercise system requires an almost Zero Footprint Workout™ environment, and it can be either self-resisted, use a variety of readily available improvised equipment, or a pair of inexpensive yet amazingly effective Iso-Bows™. Whatever you choose to use, as long as you apply the right amount of force, good technique, and follow the basic best practice rules of sensible exercise, then you can expect to benefit from a high-intensity professional-level workout.

Furthermore, with the isometric exercise system, it is possible to complete an advanced 18-exercise total-body workout routine in as little as only 126 seconds, or in exchange for just 2 minutes and 6 seconds out of your working day. Furthermore, even a total-body workout session can be completed without ever leaving the desk or workstation. The positive benefits gained from between just 49 seconds and 126 seconds of exercise are enormous for both the business and the person.

Even if only the 7 basic exercises we took from "The 70 Second Difference™" book were performed, the result is still a basic total-body workout session. 7 exercises taking just 7 seconds to perform is just 49 seconds in total. Even by adding 20 seconds of rest time to each of the 7-second exercises, it will still only take a total of 189 seconds to complete a total-body workout.

More importantly, over the course of a working day, it is easily possible to perform one exercise either every half hour or even every hour if you are exceptionally busy. The fact is that performing a workout lasting just 49 seconds spread out over a working day would not even be noticeable. There would be zero impact on any productivity time loss.

It is also clear that time is the most precious commodity that we all possess, and almost always, we never have enough of it to spare. Therefore, why waste your precious time performing massively time-consuming, inconvenient, and expensive traditional gym-based exercise sessions?

It is a truth that the majority of people in the world do not particularly enjoy exercising and given a choice they would prefer not to. However, most people know that they must do some exercise for their health, so it is a dilemma. Most coaches and gyms recommend that people perform exercise sessions that are time-consuming and require certain equipment. This becomes part of the overall problem of why most people do not exercise, or why they soon stop exercising after joining a gym in an effort to keep their New Year's resolution. Since time is so precious for most people, and since most people want to spend the minimum time and effort exercising, the isometric exercise system is the ideal solution. Is it the perfect system? No, it is not. However, no single exercise system is perfect. Does the isometric exercise system deliver excellent results in a short space of time, and is it scientifically proven? Yes, it certainly does and is.

If you are self-employed, then the benefits of the isometric exercise system are immediately clear. Saving time, money, stress, and effort all add up to giving you much more time to devote to growing your business, making money, and spending more time with your family are all excellent choices. it is just a common-sense approach, especially since the results you will get from the isometric exercise system will either be equal to or typically better than traditional gym-based sessions.

If you work for a company, then it is inconceivable that any employer would actually prefer an employee to underperform, be more stressed, less happy, less healthy, more prone to taking time off sick, for them to enjoy poorer inter-colleague relationships, and for them to deliver fewer results than they potentially could do, all for the sake of taking either a minimum of 49 seconds or a maximum of 126 seconds out of the working day.

In our opinion, it would be nothing short of utter stupidity for any employer/company leadership not to openly embrace the isometric system which enables employees to Workout at Work™.

What is TWiEA™?

For more information and member's online video resources for TWiEA members, visit www.TWiEA.com. TWiEA™ is the acronym for The World Isometric Exercise Association which is the governing body for all types of isometric exercise. Its mission is to help set and maintain standards of excellence in teaching and promoting all types of isometric exercise. TWiEA™ seeks to ensure that scientifically proven isometric exercise techniques are taught as part of an integrated overall approach to the total-body exercise solutions provided by fitness professionals. This creates a much higher probability that busy clients facing real-life time crunches can maintain an effective exercise program. Isometric exercise is every bit as effective at building muscle and strength as other traditional forms of resistance training. It is also a time-saving and money-saving exercise solution that almost anyone can perform without any special equipment.

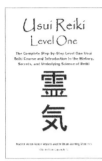

Usui Reiki Level One

A comprehensive introduction to Reiki, its history, and the science underpinning it. This course is written in an easy-to-understand step-by-step way so you will know exactly what to do and when to do it. This and other books in the series also serve as course manuals for our online or in-person Reiki students.

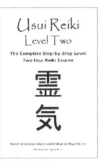

Usui Reiki Level Two

The Reiki Level Two course is the next logical step in your Reiki journey as you learn the Power Symbols and how to use them. This course is without any history or science learned in book one. It is laid out logically in an easy-to-understand step-by-step way so you will know exactly what to do and when to do it.

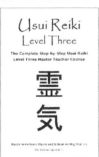

Usui Reiki Level Three

The Level Three Master Teacher course is the final step for those inspired by completing Level Two. This is a pure Level Three course without any history or science that would have been learned in book one. It is laid out logically in an easy-to-understand step-by-step way so you will know exactly what to do and when to do it.

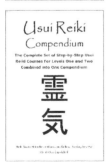

Usui Reiki Compendium – Levels One and Two

The Reiki Compendium is a combination, complete and unabridged, book of our Usui Reiki Level One and Two courses. It is ideal for those wishing to progress right through both levels of their Reiki Journey. This and other books in the series also serve as course manuals for our online or in-person Reiki Students.

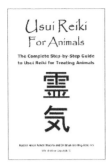

Usui Reiki for Treating Animals

The Usui Reiki for Animals book is ideal for practitioners at any level who want to learn tips and techniques for treating animals of all kinds safely and effectively. It also covers the slight differences in animal chakras and energy centres as well as others that are unique to certain animals.

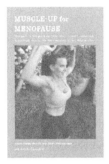

Muscle-up For Menopause

Approved by TWiEA – The World Isometric Exercise Association. Menopause cannot be avoided so take control of every element possible. Brief yet intense exercise sessions that place the minimum demand on your ability to recover combined with a high-protein plant-based diet can make all the difference between making life easier or harder during menopause. This course can be performed with or without equipment.

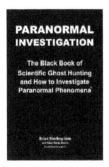

Paranormal Investigation - The Black Book of Scientific Ghost Hunting and How to Investigate Paranormal Phenomena™ This best-selling book is ideal for beginners and advanced investigators who want to apply a more scientific approach. It contains a special scientific critical path graphic page to work from and a step-by-step guide to a complete paranormal investigation. It also tells you how to protect yourself from malevolent paranormal entities.

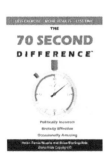

The 70 Second Difference™ - The Politically Incorrect, Occasionally Amusing, and Brutally Effective Guide to Strength, Fitness and Better Health

Approved by TWiEA – The World Isometric Exercise Association. This is a science-based no-nonsense guide about the most efficient ways to exercise, build muscle and strength, and how lifestyle and dietary choices affect you. Just 70 seconds a day of focused science-based exercise can give you a total-body workout.

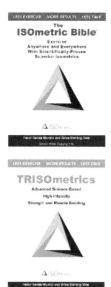

The ISOmetric Bible™ - Exercise Anywhere with Scientifically Proven Isometrics

Approved by TWiEA – The World Isometric Exercise Association. A complete, practical, scientific, and user-friendly benchmark book about scientifically proven isometric exercise. No special equipment is needed for a total-body workout.

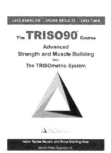

TRISOmetrics™ - Advanced Science-Based High-Intensity Strength and Muscle Building

Approved by TWiEA – The World Isometric Exercise Association. An advanced, science-based high-intensity exercise system combining 3 scientifically proven techniques into a powerful new exercise system. It can be performed with or without equipment when travelling, or as part of a gym-based exercise routine.

The TRISO90™ Course – Advanced Strength and Muscle Building with The TRISOmetrics™ System

Approved by TWiEA – The World Isometric Exercise Association. A 90-day/12-week step-by-step highly advanced bodybuilding/shaping and strength-training exercise course. It combines three proven science-based principles It can be performed with or without equipment, or as part of a gym-based exercise routine.

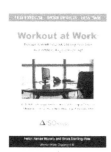

Workout at Work™ - Exercise at Work Without Anyone Even Knowing What You're Doing!

Approved by TWiEA – The World Isometric Exercise Association. Time is the #1 reason why people do not exercise. The average person spends over 10 years of their life at a desk! With scientifically proven isometric exercise, you can exercise effectively at work without ever leaving your desk.

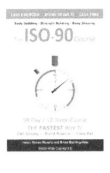

The ISO90™ Course – The 12-Week/90-Day Shape-up and Get Strong Course

Approved by TWiEA – The World Isometric Exercise Association. A complete step-by-step 90-day/12-week isometric body shaping, bodybuilding, and strength-building course ideal for both beginners and advanced.

Isometric Power Exercises for Martial Arts™ - Build Superior Strength, Muscle and Martial Arts 'Firepower' Using the Proven System Bruce Lee Used

Approved by TWiEA – The World Isometric Exercise Association. This book is a valuable resource for practical isometric exercises to build serious strength, muscle, and martial arts firepower.

Improvised Isometric Exercise Devices - The Daisy Chain - How a Simple Climber's Daisy Chain Can Become a Powerful Improvised Isometric Exercise Device or IIED

Approved by TWiEA – The World Isometric Exercise Association. Improvised Isometric Exercise Devices or IIEDs come in all shapes and sizes and are only limited by your imagination. This is a valuable resource listing practical exercises that can be performed as well as how to safely extend the daisy chain.

The Climber's Sling - How a Simple Climber's Sling Can Become a Powerful Improvised Isometric Device or IIED

Approved by TWiEA – The World Isometric Exercise Association.

IIEDs come in all shapes and sizes and are only limited by your imagination. This is a valuable resource listing practical isometric exercises that can be performed as well as how to safely extend the climber's sling.

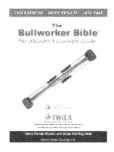

The Bullworker Bible™ The Ultimate Science-Based Guide to The Classic Personal Multi-Gym

Approved by TWiEA – The World Isometric Exercise Association. and the makers of The Bullworker. The original and best guide for all Bullworker® users and the companion book to The Bullworker 90™ Course. It is complete, science-based, and user-friendly showing how the device should be used to deliver maximum results. Also essential for the Steel Bow®.

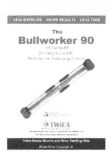

The Bullworker 90™ Course – The Ultimate Science-Based 12-Week/90-Day Get Strong and Grow Muscle Course Using the Classic Personal Multi-Gym

Approved by TWiEA – The World Isometric Exercise Association. and the makers of The Bullworker. A 90-day/12-week step-by-step course and companion book to The Bullworker Bible™. Each week has a detailed note section, so you know exactly what to do and when to do it.

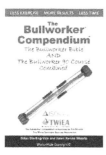

The Bullworker Compendium™ - The Bullworker Bible™ and The Bullworker90™ Course Combined

Approved by TWiEA – The World Isometric Exercise Association. and the makers of The Bullworker. The Bullworker Compendium™ combines both The Bullworker Bible™ and The Bullworker 90™ Course in a single huge book.

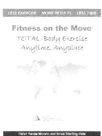

Fitness on the Move™ - Enjoy Gym-Quality Workout Sessions ANYWHERE! Approved by TWiEA – The World Isometric Exercise Association. This book lists practical exercises that can be performed while travelling almost anywhere and in any vehicle. If there is enough space to either sit down and/or stand upright, then you can perform a total-body workout!

237

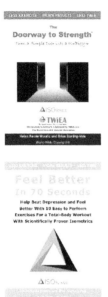

The Doorway to Strength™ - Turn a Door into a Strength-Building Multigym

Approved by TWiEA – The World Isometric Exercise Association. It shows how a simple door, doorway, and frame can be used to create a multi-gym of exercises using the amazing Iso-Bow®. Required: 2 x Iso-Bows®, a solid door and frame, and a door wedge/stop.

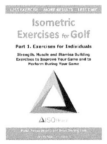

Feel Better In 70 Seconds™

Help Beat Depression and Feel Better With 10 Easy-to-Perform Exercises for a Total-Body Workout with Scientifically Proven Isometrics. Approved by TWiEA – The World Isometric Exercise Association. Research shows that exercise can help to beat depression and can be done with little or no money, time, or space. 70 seconds of consecutive exercise is all that is needed to perform a 10-exercise total-body workout routine using the scientifically proven isometric exercise system. Required: 2 x Iso-Bows®

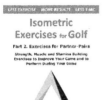

Isometric Exercises for Golf™ Part 1. Exercises for Individuals.

Approved by TWiEA – The World Isometric Exercise Association. Isometric exercises can be performed either during a game or practice and with just one exercise at each of the 18-holes then you get a total-body workout at the end of a game. The average golf club is a perfect Improvised Isometric Exercise Device or IIED. Part 1. is a resource guide of exercises for individuals with special exercises to increase the power of the swing.

Isometric Exercises for Golf™ Part 2. Partner-Pairs

Approved by TWiEA – The World Isometric Exercise Association.

The companion to Book 1 is focused on exercises that are best performed in partnered pairs during a break, a game, or during practice sessions.

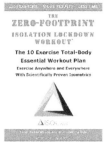

The Zero-Footprint Isolation Lockdown Workout - The 10 Exercise Total-Body Essential Workout Plan Exercise Anywhere and Everywhere with Scientifically Proven Isometrics. Approved by TWiEA – The World Isometric Exercise Association. 10 essential total-body exercises that can be performed anywhere, if you can stand and sit, then you can perform a powerful workout routine in as little as 70 seconds a day! NOTE: This is a variation of The 70 Second Difference™ workout.

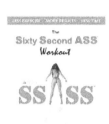

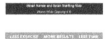

The Sixty Second ASS Workout™ - The Ultimate 60-Second Workout to Shape, Tone, Lift, and Give You the Backside You've Always Wanted. Approved by TWiEA – The World Isometric Exercise Association. The fastest and most effective "ass" workout ever devised. Scientifically proven exercises deliver a no-nonsense time-efficient workout.

Isometric Exercises for Nordic Walking and Trekking™ - Part 1. Exercises for Individuals. Approved by TWiEA – The World Isometric Exercise Association. Perform gym-quality total-body isometric exercise routines during walk breaks almost anywhere using walking/trekking poles as an IIED or Improvised Isometric Exercise Device. Book 1. is a resource guide of exercises performed by individuals.

Isometric Exercises for Nordic Walking and Trekking™ - Part 2. Exercises for Walk Partner-Pairs
Approved by TWiEA – The World Isometric Exercise Association.
This is the companion to Book 1 and is focused on exercises that are best performed as a partner-pair, with a friend.

239

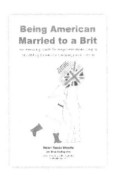

Being American Married to a Brit™ - An Amusing Guide for Anglo-American Couples Divided by a Common Language and Culture

A quirky, eye-opening, and fun-filled roller-coaster ride of how even the most basic everyday transatlantic conversations can bring laughter. It is dedicated to all transatlantic couples who are divided and confused by their common language.

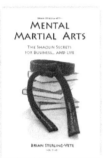

Mental Martial Arts™ - intellectual Life and Business Combat Skills

A system of intellectual languages and life-combat skills using the tactics and principles of physical martial arts. Learn how to verbally, and intellectually guide, channel, and redirect the energy of powerful people, and large organisations to achieve the outcomes that you desire.

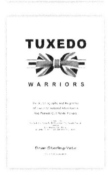

Tuxedo Warriors™

The companion book to both The Tuxedo Warrior book and movie is the biography and autobiography of the iconic cult author, composer, and moviemaker Cliff Twemlow. It continues the story from where Cliff's book finishes and it is the most complete biography of Cliff Twemlow ever written. It is also the autobiography of Brian Sterling-Vete.

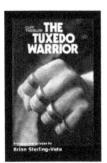

The Tuxedo Warrior™ by Cliff Twemlow – Prologue and epilogue by Brian Sterling-Vete.

There are many ways in which a Doorman can gain respect. Numerous methods were applied to the principle. In my profession, every available technique must be utilised, depending on the situation and circumstances. Would-be transgressors either move off the premises and quietly acknowledge your diplomatic approach. Or, the other alternative whereby physical persuasion must be exercised, which either quells their pugilistic desires or it triggers their aggressive instincts, turning the whole incident into a bloody and violent encounter. 'The Tuxedo Warrior,' pulls no punches in its brawling, savage, colourful, and entertaining exposure of society's nightlife activities.

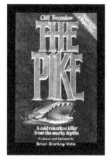

The Pike™ by Cliff Twemlow – Prologue and epilogue by Brian Sterling-Vete.
ITS FIRST VICTIMS - A screeching swan... A fisherman overboard... A drunken woman...
One by one, the mysterious killer in Lake Windermere claims its terrified victims. Tearing off limbs with its monstrous teeth, horribly mutilating bodies. Fear sweeps the peaceful holiday resort when experts identify the creature as a giant pike.... A hellish creature with the strength to rupture boats, and the anger to attack them. But for some, the terror becomes a bonanza—the traders who cater to the gathering crowds of ghouls on the shore. And they will do anything to stop divers from finding the creature. Meanwhile, the ripples of bloodshed widen.... The Pike.

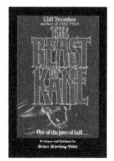

The Beast of Kane™ by Cliff Twemlow – Prologue and epilogue by Brian Sterling-Vete.
When the Gordon Family open their door to a stray Elkhound, they unwittingly welcome in the forces of evil. For, according to the local priest, the huge dog is Satan himself, fulfilling an ancient prophecy. But no one will believe this warning... Even when sheep – and wolves – are mysteriously slaughtered. Even when frenzied pets turn on their owners. Even when Emily Forrest is savagely eaten alive – the first of many human victims. As winter tightens its icy grip on the remote town of Kane, its unprotected people must face an unearthly terror.

241

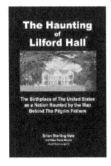

The Haunting of Lilford Hall™ - The Birthplace of the United States as a Nation Haunted by the Man Behind The Pilgrim Fathers. This is one of the most baffling cases ever recorded of paranormal activity experienced by multiple people between 2012 and 2013. Robert Browne is the man responsible for getting the Pilgrim Fathers to sail on The Mayflower in 1620 and it is believed that his ghost still haunts Lilford Hall.

Paranormal Dictionary

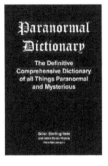

A complete and comprehensive guide to all of the most common paranormal terminology, entities, and equipment used during investigations, plus, a few enduring mysteries for good measure. It is ideal for both new and experienced investigators.

Made in United States
North Haven, CT
20 February 2024

48912237R00134